Doctor, Why Can't I Lose Weight?

A Doctor's Simple Guide to Safe, Sustainable Weight Loss

Dr Prabhat Das

MD, PhD, ACP

Better Health with Dr Das Series

Disclaimer
This book is intended solely for educational and informational purposes. It is not meant to replace personal medical advice, diagnosis, or treatment. Although I am a licensed physician, reading this book does not establish a doctor–patient relationship. Each individual's health condition, medical history, and risk factors are unique. Any medical decision should be made in partnership with your own healthcare professional who understands your specific situation. Medical science is continually advancing. New research and updated guidelines may lead to changes in recommendations over time.

Paperback ISBN: 978-1-971672-08-3
eBook ISBN: 978-1-971672-09-0

Typeset in font *Garamond* by *Indica Infomedia*, New Delhi, India
Printed in the United States of America

About the Author

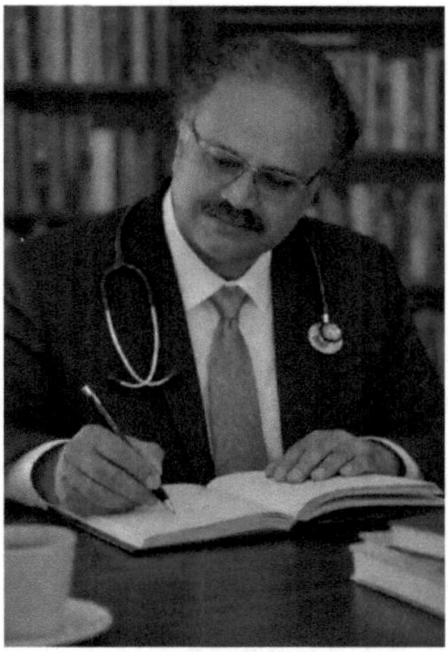

I am **Dr. Prabhat Das, MD, PhD, FACP**. My journey in medicine began in India, and for more than thirty-five years I have had the privilege of practicing medicine in the United States. I trained in **Internal Medicine, Pulmonary Diseases, and Critical Care**, and throughout these decades medicine has been far more than a career for me. It has been a lifelong calling rooted in learning, service, and deep respect for the people who place their trust in their physician.

Over the course of my medical career, I have cared for patients in many different settings. I have seen patients in my office for everyday health concerns, treated people in busy emergency rooms, managed complex illnesses in the hospital, and cared for the most critically ill patients in intensive care units. Thousands of patients have sat across from me during office visits. Many more have depended on careful decisions made during difficult and urgent moments in the hospital and ICU.

But medicine is not only about diagnoses, tests, and treatments. Every day I have listened to patients speak about their worries, their fears, their uncertainty, and often the many questions they hesitate to ask. Those conversations have taught me something profound. People want clear information, honest guidance, and reassurance they can trust. They want to understand their health so they can take better care of themselves and the people they love.

These experiences have shaped how I think about health, illness, prevention, and the deeply human side of healing.

Through the **"Better Health with Dr Das" series**, I hope to reach many individuals I may never meet personally in my office. Many people struggle quietly with health questions and confusing medical information. My goal in these books is simple. I want to explain important medical topics in a clear, practical, and reassuring way so that readers feel informed, confident, and empowered to make better decisions about their health. The information presented in these books is based on reliable scientific knowledge and decades of clinical experience.

If these books bring clarity to someone who feels confused, comfort to someone who feels worried, or practical help to someone trying to improve their health, then this effort will have been deeply worthwhile.

Helping people live healthier, better informed lives continues to be one of the greatest privileges and satisfactions of my professional life.

Table of Contents

About the Author 5

Chapter 1: Why Can't I Lose Weight? 13

Chapter 2: What Is Obesity, and Why Does It Matter? 29

Chapter 3: How Obesity Develops 39

Chapter 4: Why Weight Loss Is So Difficult 51

Chapter 5: Diet and Eating Patterns: A Practical, Sustainable Approach 61

Chapter 6: Behavior Change and Habit Formation 75

Chapter 7: Psychological Factors and Emotional Eating 87

Chapter 8: Physical Activity and Exercise: A Realistic Approach 101

Chapter 9: When Is Medical Treatment Needed? 113

Chapter 10: Weight Loss Medications: What You Should Know 123

Chapter 11: GLP-1 Medications: A New Era in Weight Loss 133

Chapter 12: Weight Loss Surgery: An Important Option for Some 143

Chapter 13: Preventing Weight Regain: Protecting Your Progress 153

Chapter 14: Your Long-Term Strategy for Lifelong Weight Control 165

Preface

Over the past several decades of practicing medicine, I have had the privilege of caring for thousands of patients. I have seen people come to my office with a wide range of concerns, but one topic comes up again and again -Weight.

Sometimes it is discussed openly.

Sometimes it is mentioned hesitantly.

And sometimes, it is not spoken at all, but it is clearly present in the patient's mind.

I have met individuals who are intelligent, disciplined, and hardworking, yet deeply frustrated with their inability to lose weight. Many have tried multiple diets, exercise plans, and programs. Some have seen temporary success, only to regain the weight later. Others feel stuck, discouraged, and unsure of what to do next.

Weight gain and weight loss are not simple processes. They are influenced by many factors, including biology, habits, emotions, environment, sleep, stress, and medical conditions. When all of these come together, the challenge becomes much more complex than most people expect.

Through this book, I want to speak to you the same way I speak to my patients in my office, calmly, honestly, and with genuine concern for your well-being.

My goal is not to offer quick fixes or unrealistic promises. You will not find extreme diets or miracle solutions here. This book is written in simple language, without unnecessary complexity, so that you can clearly understand what is happening in your body and what you can do about it.

The purpose of this book is not to judge you. It is to support you. Change does not happen overnight. It happens step by step, through understanding, consistency, and patience.

With sincere good wishes for your health and well-being,

Dr Prabhat Das, MD, PhD

Chapter 1

Why Can't I Lose Weight?

If you have ever stood on a scale and felt your heart sink, you are not alone.

If you have ever promised yourself that this time would be different, only to find yourself slipping back into old habits after a few days or a few weeks, you are not alone either.

And if you have ever asked in frustration, sadness, or quiet disbelief, "Why can't I lose weight?" then this chapter is meant for you.

Over many years of medical practice, I have heard this question again and again. People ask it in different ways, but the pain behind the question is often the same. Some ask with irritation. Some with shame. Some with deep tiredness. Some ask almost in a whisper, as if they are admitting a personal failure. Many have already tried several diets, exercise plans, or weight loss programs. They have lost a few pounds, gained them back, and then blamed themselves. After repeating this cycle enough times, many begin to believe that they simply do not have what it takes.

That belief is often wrong.

One of the most important things I want to tell you at the beginning of this book is this: if you have struggled with weight for years, it does not automatically mean that you are lazy, weak, careless, or lacking in discipline. Weight gain and weight loss are far more complicated than most people are led to believe. The human body is not a simple machine. It is a living, adapting system shaped by biology, environment, habits, emotions, sleep, stress, age, medications, hormones, and life circumstances. When all of those forces push in the wrong direction, losing weight can become far more difficult than it appears from the outside.

That is why so many intelligent, sincere, responsible people continue to struggle.

This book is not here to shame you. It is here to help you understand what is really happening and what can truly help. My goal is not to offer magical promises or empty motivation. My goal is to explain the problem clearly, honestly, and compassionately, so that you can begin to see your own struggle in a better light. Once you understand why this problem happens, why it is so persistent, and why the body often fights against weight loss, you can begin to approach it in a wiser and more realistic way.

That is where meaningful change begins.

A Struggle Shared by Millions

One of the cruelest parts of weight problems is that they often feel deeply personal. A person may look around and assume that everyone else has figured something out that they have not. They may feel embarrassed in restaurants, uncomfortable at family gatherings, uneasy during doctor visits, and self-conscious when buying clothes. Some begin avoiding mirrors. Others avoid photographs. Some stop attending social events because they do not feel comfortable in their own body.

Yet the truth is that this struggle is extremely common.

Millions of people are dealing with the same issue. They may not talk about it openly, but they are carrying the same disappointment, the same frustration, and the same questions. In many cases, they are living in conditions that quietly promote weight gain every day. Food is everywhere. Portions are larger than they used to be. Highly processed foods are cheap, convenient, heavily advertised, and engineered to be appealing. Many people sit for long hours at work. Many are tired when they come home. Sleep is often poor. Stress is constant. Daily schedules are crowded. Under these conditions, slow weight gain becomes very easy.

A person may gain only a few pounds a year and hardly notice it. But over ten or fifteen years, those few pounds quietly accumulate. One day, the person looks at an old photograph or sees a new number on the scale and feels shocked. The weight did not appear overnight, but the realization can still feel sudden and painful.

That slow, silent progression is one reason obesity can feel so discouraging. By the time the problem becomes obvious, it may already feel deeply rooted.

Why Simple Advice Often Fails

Most people have heard the standard advice: eat less and move more.

At one level, this advice sounds reasonable. Yes, food intake matters. Yes, physical activity matters. But when that advice is presented as if the whole problem is simple, it leaves out too much of the truth.

If weight loss were only a matter of hearing the correct advice, far fewer people would be struggling.

The real problem is that the body and the mind do not always cooperate with good intentions. A person may start with enthusiasm, cut down portions, skip snacks, go walking, and do everything they can to follow the plan. At first, a few pounds may come off. Then hunger grows stronger. Cravings become more intense. Energy drops. Progress slows. The scale stops moving. Discouragement begins. The person starts to feel deprived, tired, and mentally worn out. Then one stressful week, one holiday, one emotional setback, or one moment of exhaustion pulls them back toward old habits.

When that happens, many people conclude that they failed because they did not try hard enough.

But often the deeper truth is that they were fighting against a much more complex problem than they understood.

It Is Not Just About Willpower

This may be one of the most important lessons in the entire book.

Obesity is not simply a failure of willpower.

Willpower has a role. Choices matter. Habits matter. Personal responsibility matters. But if we treat willpower as the whole explanation, we misunderstand the problem and we make people feel unnecessarily ashamed.

I have seen many patients who are extremely disciplined in other parts of life. They work long hours, care for family members, manage responsibilities, and function under pressure. These are not weak people. Yet they still struggle with weight. That alone should tell us that something more complicated is going on.

The body has powerful systems designed to protect itself from perceived starvation. When you lose weight, the body often responds by increasing hunger and reducing the number of calories it burns. In simple terms, the body begins to resist. It tries to pull you back toward your former weight. At the same time, your mind becomes more aware of food. Tempting foods seem harder to resist. Cravings become more frequent. Emotional eating may return. Habits that had been controlled for weeks begin to creep back in.

This is why weight loss can feel like a battle that becomes harder over time instead of easier.

Understanding this does not remove personal responsibility. But it does replace unfair blame with a more accurate picture.

The Many Forces That Shape Body Weight

Weight is influenced by a wide range of factors, and these factors often interact with one another.

Genetics

Some people are naturally more likely to gain weight than others. Genetics can affect appetite, satiety, metabolism, body fat distribution, and the body's tendency to store energy. This does not mean that weight problems are fully predetermined. It does mean that some people are starting the race with a heavier burden.

Environment

Modern life constantly pushes people toward overeating and inactivity. Tempting foods are easy to find. Portions are oversized. Social life often revolves around food. Sedentary work has become common. By the end of the day, many people are too tired to cook, exercise, or think carefully about food choices.

Sleep

Poor sleep can quietly damage weight control. When you are sleep-deprived, hunger often increases, cravings become stronger, and the desire for sugary or high-calorie foods rises. At the same time, fatigue makes movement less appealing.

Stress

Stress affects eating in powerful ways. Some people lose appetite under stress, but many do the opposite. They eat more, snack more, crave comfort foods, and lose control more easily. Stress also worsens sleep and drains energy, creating a double burden.

Hormones and Medical Factors

Certain medical conditions and medications can contribute to weight gain or make weight loss harder. Hormonal problems, insulin resistance, steroids, some antidepressants, and other medicines can all play a role. This is one reason medical evaluation can be important in some cases.

Age and Life Circumstances

As people grow older, muscle mass tends to decline unless it is actively maintained. Daily movement may decrease. Busy careers, family life, emotional losses, illness, and social changes all influence eating and activity patterns. Weight that was once easy to control may become much harder to manage.

Habits and Emotions

Many people eat for reasons that have little to do with hunger. They eat because they are stressed, lonely, bored, sad, tired, or simply following a familiar routine. Over time, those repeated patterns become deeply rooted habits, and habits can feel almost automatic.

When these forces come together, the struggle becomes much easier to understand.

Why Repeated Dieting Often Leaves People Defeated

By the time many people seek real help, they have already tried multiple diets. Some have tried low-fat diets, low-carbohydrate diets, juice plans, meal replacements, fasting plans, packaged foods, weight loss pills, online advice, and expensive commercial programs. Almost all of them began with hope.

Many of those efforts produced some short-term success. But that success often faded.

The reason is not always lack of effort. Often the method itself was flawed. Some plans are too strict. Some are too joyless. Some ignore hunger, emotional eating, family life, social life, work schedules, or simple human nature. Some are built for rapid short-term loss, not long-term maintenance. Others are so unrealistic that no ordinary person could sustain them for months, let alone years.

When such plans fail, people rarely blame the plan. They blame themselves.

That is tragic, because repeated discouragement can slowly destroy confidence. A person begins each new attempt with less hope than before. They start expecting failure even before they begin.

That emotional exhaustion is real, and it deserves to be recognized.

The Hidden Emotional Weight

Excess body weight places stress on the body, but it also places a burden on the mind.

Many people living with obesity carry an invisible load of guilt, shame, self-criticism, and disappointment. They may feel judged by strangers, dismissed by doctors, misunderstood by family members, or trapped in a body that no longer feels like their own. Some begin to think that every problem in life is somehow connected to their weight. Others feel they have lost control, and with that loss comes a deep sense of discouragement.

These feelings can become part of the cycle.

A person feels upset, stressed, or ashamed. They turn to food for comfort. The eating brings temporary relief. Then guilt returns. That guilt adds to emotional pain, and emotional pain often leads back to eating. Over time, this cycle can become hard to break.

That is why weight is never only a nutritional issue. It is often emotional, behavioral, biological, and social all at once.

Real progress begins when we stop treating obesity like a simple moral failure and start seeing it as a complex human problem.

A Different Way of Looking at Success

Another reason people feel defeated is that they often define success too narrowly.

Many imagine that weight loss only counts if they reach an ideal number on the scale. If they lose some weight but not all of it, they may feel they have failed. If they improve health but still want to lose more, they may overlook how far they have already come.

But this way of thinking is both discouraging and inaccurate.

In medicine, even modest weight loss can matter. Losing 5 to 10 percent of body weight can improve blood pressure, blood sugar, joint pain, sleep quality, energy level, and overall health. A person who is moving better, breathing better, sleeping better, and feeling stronger is making real progress even if the journey is not complete.

Health improvement matters. Better habits matter. Increased self-awareness matters. Greater control over eating matters. Learning how your body and mind respond to food matters.

The journey does not have to be perfect to be meaningful.

What This Book Will Try to Do

This book will not promise miracles.

It will not tell you that one special food, one popular diet, one injection, or one trick will solve everything. It will not ask you to become perfect. It will not ask you to hate yourself into change.

Instead, it will try to do something more useful.

It will help you understand what obesity really is. It will explain how weight gain develops, why the body resists weight loss, how excess weight affects health, and why the struggle is often much harder than it appears. It will discuss food, habits, emotional eating, behavior change, physical activity, medicines, GLP-1 drugs, surgical options, and long-term maintenance. Most importantly, it will keep returning to one central idea: lasting improvement comes from understanding the problem clearly and approaching it with realism, patience, and persistence.

This is not a book about chasing perfection.

It is a book about making wiser choices, building better patterns, and creating a more sustainable path forward.

You Are Not Starting from Nothing

If you have tried and failed before, it is easy to feel that you are back at the beginning.

But you are not.

You are beginning from experience.

Your past attempts, even the unsuccessful ones, have taught you something. They have shown you what triggers overeating, what kinds of plans are too strict, what situations break your routine, what emotional states affect your eating, what times of day are most dangerous, and what helps even a little. Those lessons matter.

The mistake is not that you have tried before.

The mistake would be ignoring what those attempts have already taught you.

A wiser plan is built not on shame, but on honest reflection.

Hope, But Not False Hope

Some readers may be tired of encouragement. They have heard too many promises before. They do not want more empty words.

I understand that.

So let me be clear. Weight loss is often difficult. It may be slow. It may be uneven. There may be plateaus, setbacks, and disappointment along the way. For many people, long-term maintenance is harder than the first few weeks of losing weight. There is no single method that works for everyone.

But meaningful improvement is possible.

People do learn to eat differently. People do become more active. People do reduce emotional eating. People do improve their sleep, their blood pressure, their diabetes, and their quality of life. Some benefit from behavior change alone. Some need medication. Some do well with GLP-1 treatment. Some need surgery. Many people improve in ways that once felt impossible.

The path may not be quick or simple, but real progress can happen.

Hope is most useful when it is honest, grounded, and joined with a practical plan.

An Invitation to Begin Differently

This chapter is not asking you to begin a punishing new diet tonight.

It is not asking you to erase the past.

It is not asking you to become someone else overnight.

It is simply inviting you to look at your weight struggle with more honesty and less self-blame.

It is inviting you to stop seeing obesity as a character flaw.

It is inviting you to understand that this is a complex medical and behavioral problem, one that deserves thoughtful care, not shame.

And it is inviting you to take the next step with a little more patience, a little more wisdom, and a little more hope.

In the chapters ahead, we will go deeper into the science, the habits, the emotions, the treatments, and the strategies that matter most. By the end of this book, my hope is that you will not only understand your struggle more clearly, but also feel more capable of doing something about it.

That is how lasting change begins.

Main Points to Remember

- If you struggle with weight, you are far from alone.

- Obesity is not simply a problem of weak willpower.
- Weight is influenced by biology, environment, sleep, stress, emotions, habits, age, medications, and life circumstances.
- Many diets fail because they are too strict, unrealistic, or hard to sustain.
- The body often fights against weight loss by increasing hunger and reducing energy use.
- Weight problems affect emotional wellbeing as well as physical health.
- Even modest weight loss can lead to meaningful health improvement.
- Past failures do not mean you are hopeless. They can teach you valuable lessons.
- Real progress usually comes from understanding the problem better and choosing a long-term, realistic approach.

What You Can Do Now

Before moving to the next chapter, take a little time to reflect on your own story. Write your answers down if possible. A notebook can be very helpful.

1. Look back at your weight history

Ask yourself:

- When did your weight start to rise?

- Was it gradual or sudden?
- Were certain life events connected to weight gain, such as stress, illness, aging, grief, family pressure, pregnancy, poor sleep, or a sedentary job?

2. List your past weight loss attempts

Write down:

- What you tried
- What seemed to help
- What made the plan hard to continue
- What happened after you stopped

3. Identify your main barriers

Be honest with yourself. Common barriers include:

- Constant hunger
- Cravings
- Stress eating
- Late-night eating
- Fatigue
- Poor sleep
- Busy schedule
- Lack of exercise
- Emotional struggles
- Repeated discouragement

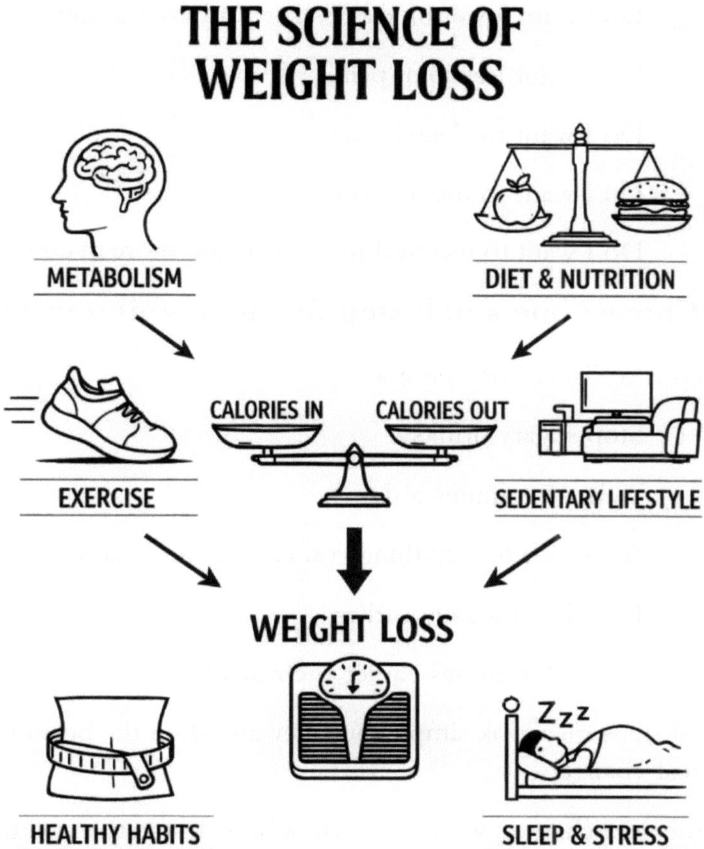
THE SCIENCE OF WEIGHT LOSS
METABOLISM
DIET & NUTRITION
EXERCISE
CALORIES IN
CALORIES OUT
SEDENTARY LIFESTYLE
WEIGHT LOSS
Zzz
HEALTHY HABITS
SLEEP & STRESS

4. Clarify why you want to lose weight

Try to go deeper than appearance alone. Ask:

- Do I want more energy?
- Do I want lower blood pressure or better blood sugar?
- Do I want less joint pain?
- Do I want to sleep better?
- Do I want to move more easily?
- Do I want to feel healthier, freer, and more in control?

5. Choose one small step for the coming week

Keep it realistic. For example:

- Stop sugary drinks
- Walk 15 minutes a day
- Write down everything you eat for three days
- Eat dinner a little earlier
- Sleep 30 minutes earlier each night

Small steps may look simple, but they are often the beginning of real change.

In the next chapter, we will answer a basic but very important question: **What exactly is obesity, and why does it matter so much to your health?**

Chapter 2

What Is Obesity, and Why Does It Matter?

When I sit across from patients in my office and we begin talking about weight, I often notice a quiet uncertainty.

Some say, "Doctor, I know I am overweight, but am I really obese?"

Others ask, "Is this just about how I look, or is it something more serious?"

And a few simply wonder, without saying it aloud, "Is this really a medical problem?"

These are important questions. And before we talk about how to lose weight, we must first understand what we are dealing with.

Because unless we understand the problem clearly, we cannot solve it wisely.

What Does 'Obesity' Really Mean?

In simple terms, obesity means having excess body fat that can affect your health.

It is not just about the number on the scale.

Two people may weigh the same, yet one may carry more fat and less muscle, while the other has a healthier body composition. The health risks are not determined by weight alone, but by how that weight is distributed and what it represents inside the body.

This is an important shift in thinking.

Obesity is not just about appearance. It is about biology. It is about how the body functions, how organs are affected, and how long-term health is influenced.

In modern medicine, obesity is recognized as a **chronic condition**. That means it develops over time, tends to persist, and often requires ongoing attention rather than a short-term solution.

This is very different from the way many people think about it.

How Do We Measure Obesity?

Doctors need practical tools to assess weight and related health risks. The most commonly used measure is the **Body Mass Index**, or BMI.

BMI is calculated using your height and weight. It gives a general idea of whether your weight falls within a healthy range.

BMI Categories

Category	BMI
Underweight	Less than 18.5
Normal weight	18.5 to 24.9
Overweight	25 to 29.9
Obesity (Class I)	30 to 34.9
Obesity (Class II)	35 to 39.9
Severe Obesity (Class III)	40 or higher

BMI is useful because it is simple and widely available.

But it is not perfect.

It does not distinguish between fat and muscle. A physically fit person with good muscle mass may have a higher BMI without having excess body fat. On the other hand, someone with a normal BMI may still have unhealthy fat distribution, especially around the abdomen.

So BMI is a helpful starting point, not the final answer.

Why Waist Size Matters

In many ways, waist size can tell us even more than weight.

Fat around the abdomen, often called **visceral fat**, is particularly harmful. This fat surrounds internal organs and is strongly linked to diabetes, heart disease, and metabolic problems.

As a general guideline:

- Men with a waist size above 40 inches are at increased risk
- Women with a waist size above 35 inches are at increased risk

This is a simple measurement, but it provides valuable insight.

You do not need sophisticated tests to begin understanding your health. Sometimes, a measuring tape can tell an important story.

Obesity Is More Than a Number

Numbers are helpful, but they do not define you.

Two people with the same BMI may have very different health profiles.

One may be active, energetic, and metabolically healthy.

Another may have diabetes, joint pain, fatigue, and poor sleep.

That is why we must always look at the whole person.

Obesity is not just a number. It is a condition that affects the body in many different ways.

Why Obesity Matters

This brings us to a crucial point.

Why does obesity matter?

Some people believe weight is mainly about appearance. But from a medical perspective, excess body fat affects nearly every organ system.

Let us look at this in a simple, practical way.

The Heart and Blood Vessels

Excess weight increases the workload on the heart. Over time, this can lead to high blood pressure, heart disease, and increased risk of stroke.

Blood Sugar and Diabetes

Abdominal fat interferes with how the body uses insulin. This can lead to insulin resistance and eventually type 2 diabetes.

Joints and Mobility

Extra weight places stress on joints, especially the knees and hips. This often leads to pain, reduced mobility, and difficulty with daily activities.

Sleep and Breathing

Obesity is a major cause of sleep apnea, a condition that disrupts breathing during sleep and leads to fatigue and long-term health risks.

The Liver

Fat can accumulate in the liver, leading to fatty liver disease, which may progress silently over time.

Daily Energy and Quality of Life

Even without a specific diagnosis, excess weight can reduce energy, make movement difficult, and limit enjoyment of daily life.

When you look at all of this together, it becomes clear that obesity is not a cosmetic issue. It is a health issue.

Even Small Weight Loss Makes a Difference

At this point, many people feel overwhelmed.

But there is something very encouraging you should understand.

You do not need to lose all excess weight to improve your health.

Even a modest weight loss, about 5 to 10 percent of your body weight, can lead to meaningful improvements:

- Better blood pressure
- Improved blood sugar
- Less strain on joints
- Better sleep
- Increased energy

This is very important.

Progress does not have to be dramatic to be valuable.

A More Realistic Way to Think About Obesity

Once you begin to understand obesity as a chronic condition, your mindset begins to change.

Instead of expecting a quick fix, you begin to think in terms of long-term management.

Just like:

- Blood pressure needs ongoing control
- Diabetes requires continuous care

Weight management also requires ongoing attention.

This is not discouraging. It is realistic.

And realistic thinking leads to better results.

Looking Ahead

Now that we understand what obesity is and why it matters, we are ready to go deeper.

In the next chapter, we will explore an important question:

How does obesity develop over time, and why does it become so difficult to reverse?

Understanding that will help you see your own situation more clearly.

Main Points to Remember

- Obesity means excess body fat that affects health, not just body weight
- It is a chronic condition that develops over time
- BMI is useful but has limitations
- Waist size is an important indicator of risk
- Obesity affects the heart, blood sugar, joints, sleep, and liver

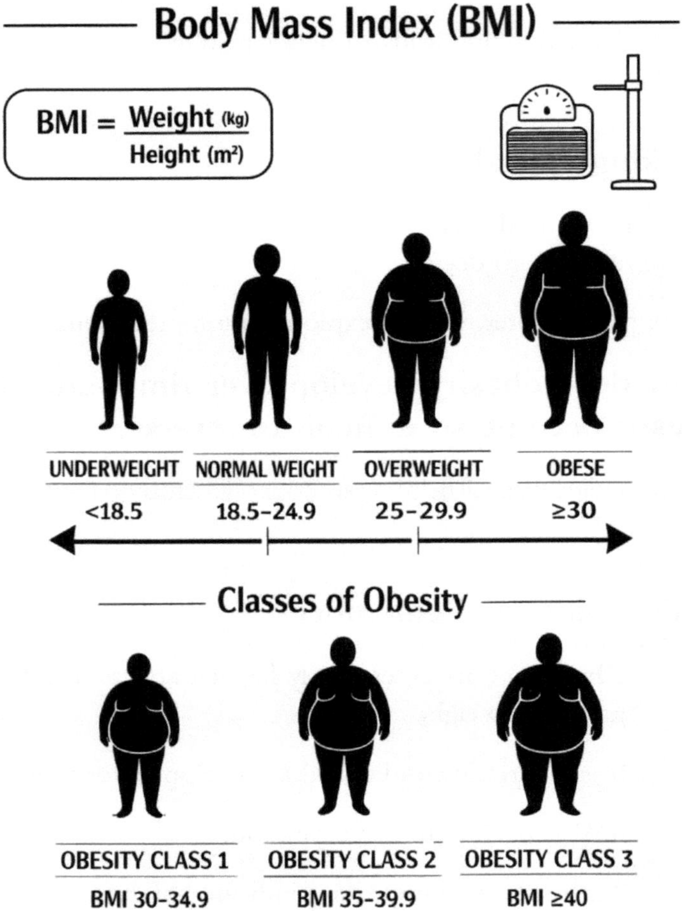
Body Mass Index (BMI)
BMI = Weight (kg) / Height (m²)
UNDERWEIGHT
<18.5
NORMAL WEIGHT
18.5–24.9
OVERWEIGHT
25–29.9
OBESE
≥30
Classes of Obesity
OBESITY CLASS 1
BMI 30–34.9
OBESITY CLASS 2
BMI 35–39.9
OBESITY CLASS 3
BMI ≥40

- It also impacts energy and quality of life
- Even modest weight loss can improve health
- Long-term management is usually needed

What You Can Do Now

Take a few simple steps to understand your starting point.

1. Check your current status

- Measure your weight and height
- Calculate your BMI
- Measure your waist size

2. Reflect honestly

Without judgment, ask yourself:

- How is my energy level?
- Do I have any weight-related health issues?

3. Write it down

Recording your current status helps you see your progress later.

4. Set a simple goal

For now, focus on awareness, not change.

5. Stay open-minded

You are not here to criticize yourself. You are here to understand.

Chapter 3
How Obesity Develops

Most people do not gain a large amount of weight all at once.

It happens quietly.

A few pounds here, a few pounds there. Clothes feel slightly tighter. Energy seems a little lower. But life is busy, and these small changes are easy to ignore. Months pass. Years pass. Then one day, the number on the scale feels surprising, even shocking.

And the question naturally follows:

"How did this happen?"

To answer that honestly, we need to understand something very important.

Weight gain is rarely caused by a single reason. It develops gradually through many small influences working together over time.

The Simple Idea That Becomes Complicated

At a basic level, weight is influenced by energy balance.

If you take in more calories than your body uses, weight tends to increase. If you use more than you take in, weight tends to decrease.

That is the simple explanation.

But real life is not simple.

Calories are not just numbers. They are affected by hunger, hormones, habits, emotions, sleep, stress, and environment. Two people can eat the same foods and have very different outcomes.

So while energy balance is true, it is not the whole story.

Small Daily Excess Adds Up

One of the most important ideas to understand is this:

Weight gain often comes from small, repeated excesses over time.

An extra 100 or 150 calories a day may not seem significant. It could be a sugary drink, a small snack, or slightly larger portions. But over months and years, this small excess adds up.

At the same time, daily activity often decreases:

- Less walking
- More sitting
- Less physical effort at work

- More screen time

When these two changes occur together, even gradually, weight gain becomes very likely.

The Modern Environment Works Against Us

We are living in a time when gaining weight has become easier than ever.

Food is:

- Easily available
- Highly processed
- Designed to be appealing
- Often rich in sugar and fat

Portion sizes have increased. Eating outside the home has become more common. Meals are often rushed or distracted.

At the same time, physical activity has decreased.

Many people spend long hours sitting at work, then come home tired, with little energy for exercise. Convenience has replaced movement in many parts of daily life.

This environment quietly pushes the body toward weight gain.

Genetics: The Starting Point Is Not the Same for Everyone

Some people gain weight more easily than others.

This is not imagination. It reflects genetic differences.

Genetics can influence:

- Appetite
- Satiety
- Fat storage
- Metabolism

If obesity runs in a family, it may reflect both shared biology and shared lifestyle patterns.

But this is important to understand clearly.

Genetics may increase the tendency to gain weight, but it does not make change impossible. It simply means that some individuals need to be more mindful and consistent.

Hormones and Body Regulation

The body uses hormones to regulate hunger, fullness, and energy use.

When these signals work well, they help maintain balance.

But when they are disrupted, problems begin.

You may feel:

- Hungry more often
- Less satisfied after eating
- Drawn toward high-calorie foods

Certain medical conditions can also affect weight, including:

- Thyroid disorders
- Insulin resistance
- Other hormonal imbalances

In addition, metabolism is not fixed. It changes with age, activity, illness, and weight itself.

Sleep: An Often Ignored Factor

Sleep plays a surprisingly important role in weight.

When sleep is inadequate:

- Hunger signals increase
- Fullness signals decrease
- Cravings for unhealthy foods increase
- Energy levels fall

A tired person is more likely to eat impulsively and less likely to stay active.

Over time, poor sleep becomes a quiet contributor to weight gain.

Stress and the Need for Comfort

Stress affects eating behavior in powerful ways.

When people feel overwhelmed, anxious, or emotionally

drained, many turn to food for comfort. This is a very human response.

Certain foods can provide temporary relief. They can create a brief sense of calm or satisfaction. But this effect does not last.

Afterward, there is often regret, followed by more stress.

This creates a cycle:

- Stress leads to eating
- Eating provides short relief
- Relief is followed by guilt
- Guilt increases stress

Breaking this cycle requires awareness, not blame.

Habits Become Automatic

Much of what we eat is not based on hunger.

It is based on habit.

People often eat:

- At the same time every day
- While watching television
- During social situations
- Out of boredom

Over time, these behaviors become automatic.

A person may reach for food without even thinking about it. These patterns can be difficult to change because they operate in the background.

But once recognized, they can be modified.

Medications and Medical Factors

Some people gain weight partly because of medications.

These may include:

- Certain antidepressants
- Steroids
- Some diabetes medications
- Other commonly used drugs

In these cases, weight gain is not simply a matter of choice.

This is why discussing weight concerns with a physician is important. Sometimes adjustments can be made.

Aging and Life Changes

As we get older, the body changes.

- Muscle mass gradually decreases
- Activity levels often decline
- Metabolism may slow

In addition, life circumstances change:

- Careers become more demanding
- Family responsibilities increase
- Time for self-care becomes limited

All of these factors can contribute to gradual weight gain.

When Everything Comes Together

Each of these factors alone may seem small.

But together, they create a powerful effect.

A person with a genetic tendency, living in a high-calorie environment, sleeping poorly, dealing with stress, following habitual eating patterns, and becoming less active over time is very likely to gain weight.

This is why obesity is not a simple problem.

It is the result of many influences acting together over many years.

A Better Way to Think About Your Situation

Instead of asking,

"What is wrong with me?"

A more helpful question is,

"What factors in my life are contributing to my weight?"

This shift in thinking is important.

It replaces blame with understanding.

And understanding allows change.

Change Begins with Awareness

You may not be able to change everything at once.

But you can begin to notice:

- When you eat
- Why you eat
- How active you are
- How you sleep
- How stress affects you

This awareness is the first step toward change.

Small adjustments, repeated consistently, can gradually shift the balance.

That is how meaningful progress begins.

Looking Ahead

Now that we understand how weight gain develops, we are ready to explore another important question:

Why does the body resist weight loss, and why does it feel so difficult to keep the weight off?

Understanding that will help you approach weight loss with

more patience and a more realistic plan.

Main Points to Remember

- Weight gain usually develops gradually over time
- Small daily excesses can lead to significant weight gain
- Modern lifestyle makes weight gain easier
- Genetics influence susceptibility but do not determine outcome
- Hormones, sleep, and stress all affect body weight
- Habits play a major role in eating behavior
- Medications and aging can contribute to weight gain
- Obesity results from multiple interacting factors
- Understanding your personal factors helps guide change

What You Can Do Now

1. Identify your main contributors

Ask yourself:

- Am I eating more than I realize?
- Am I physically inactive?
- Is my sleep poor?
- Do I eat under stress?

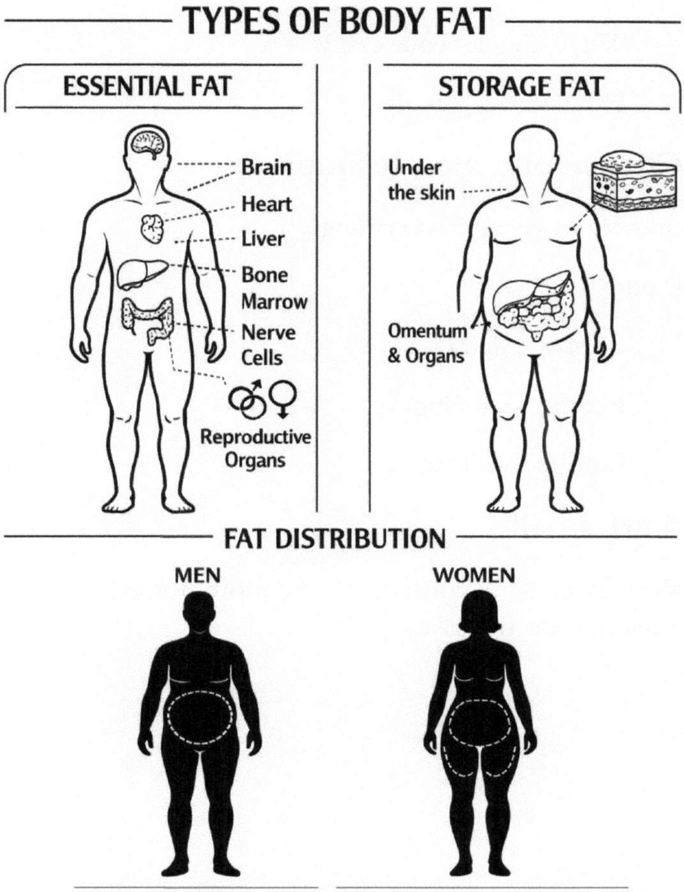
TYPES OF BODY FAT
ESSENTIAL FAT
Brain
Heart
Liver
Bone Marrow
Nerve Cells
Reproductive Organs
STORAGE FAT
Under the skin
Omentum & Organs
FAT DISTRIBUTION
MEN
WOMEN
ANDROID (VISCERAL) FAT
BMI 30-34.9
GYNOID (SUBCUTANEOUS) FAT
BMI ≥40

2. Observe your routine

For a few days, simply notice:

- When you eat
- What triggers your eating
- How active you are

3. Choose one area to improve

Do not try to change everything.

Pick one:

- Improve sleep
- Reduce snacking
- Increase walking

4. Start small

Small changes done consistently are more powerful than large changes that do not last.

Chapter 4
Why Weight Loss Is So Difficult

By now, you may be beginning to see your weight struggle in a new light.

You understand that weight gain develops slowly, influenced by many factors. But an equally important question remains:

Why is it so hard to lose weight, even when you are trying seriously?

Many people begin with strong motivation. They make changes, reduce portions, avoid certain foods, and increase activity. For a few weeks, things seem to improve. Then something changes.

Hunger increases. Energy drops. Cravings become stronger. The scale slows down or stops moving.

And frustration begins.

Patients often tell me,

"Doctor, I was doing everything right. Then it just stopped working."

This experience is extremely common.

And it is not your imagination.

Your Body Is Trying to Protect You

One of the most important truths to understand is this:

Your body does not like losing weight.

From the body's perspective, weight loss can be interpreted as a threat.

Throughout human history, food scarcity was a real danger. The body developed systems to protect against starvation. These systems are still active today.

When you start losing weight, the body reacts.

It tries to:

- Increase hunger
- Reduce energy use
- Preserve stored fat

This response is not a defect. It is a survival mechanism.

But in today's world, where excess weight is common, this natural response works against your goals.

Hunger Becomes Stronger

After weight loss begins, hunger signals often increase.

You may notice:

- Thinking about food more often
- Feeling less satisfied after meals
- Cravings becoming more intense

This is not simply a lack of discipline.

It reflects real biological changes.

Hormones that regulate hunger and fullness shift in a way that encourages you to eat more. The body is trying to restore what it has lost.

Metabolism Slows Down

Another important change happens quietly.

As you lose weight, your body needs fewer calories. That part is expected.

But in many cases, the body goes a step further.

It becomes more efficient and burns fewer calories than expected. This is sometimes called a metabolic adaptation.

In simple terms:

- You are eating less
- But your body is also using less

This makes further weight loss slower and more difficult.

The Plateau Effect

Many people experience a plateau.

At first, weight decreases. Then it stabilizes.

This can feel very discouraging.

But it often reflects the balance between:

- Reduced calorie intake
- Reduced energy expenditure

The body has adjusted.

Progress does not stop forever, but it often slows, and further effort may be needed to continue.

The Brain and Food Reward

Food is not only about energy.

It is also about pleasure.

Certain foods, especially those high in sugar, fat, and salt, stimulate reward centers in the brain. They can create a strong sense of satisfaction, even comfort.

When you try to reduce these foods, the brain notices.

Cravings may increase. Food may become more tempting. The desire for certain tastes becomes stronger.

This is one reason why simply "cutting out" foods can be difficult to sustain.

Emotional Eating Returns

During stressful or emotional periods, many people turn back to familiar eating patterns.

Even if you were doing well for weeks, one difficult day can bring back old habits.

This does not mean you have failed.

It means those patterns are still present and need to be understood and managed.

Fatigue and Mental Exhaustion

Weight loss efforts require attention and effort.

Planning meals, controlling portions, avoiding temptation, and staying active all require energy.

Over time, mental fatigue can develop.

A person may begin to feel:

- Tired of thinking about food
- Frustrated by constant effort
- Less motivated to continue

This is very real.

Sustainable plans must account for this.

Unrealistic Expectations

Another hidden problem is expectation.

Many people expect:

- Rapid weight loss
- Continuous progress
- No setbacks

When reality does not match these expectations, discouragement follows.

But the truth is:

- Weight loss is often slow
- Progress is not always steady
- Plateaus are common

Understanding this in advance helps reduce frustration.

The "All or Nothing" Trap

A common pattern looks like this:

A person follows a plan very strictly. Then one small slip occurs. A dessert, a missed workout, or a stressful day.

Instead of correcting course, the person thinks:

"I have already failed."

This leads to:

- Giving up temporarily
- Returning to old habits

- Regaining weight

This pattern can repeat many times.

The problem is not the small slip.

The problem is how it is interpreted.

Why Old Weight Feels Like a "Set Point"

Many people feel that their body is trying to return to a previous weight.

There is some truth to this.

The body often "remembers" its higher weight and tries to defend it through:

- Increased hunger
- Reduced energy use

This makes long-term maintenance challenging.

But it does not make it impossible.

With time, consistency, and the right strategies, the body can adapt to a lower weight.

A More Realistic Understanding

When you put all of this together, weight loss becomes easier to understand.

It is not difficult because you are weak.

It is difficult because:

- Your body is adapting
- Your brain is responding
- Your habits are deeply rooted
- Your environment is challenging

This is a complex process.

And it requires a thoughtful approach.

A Better Way Forward

Instead of fighting your body, the goal is to work with it.

This means:

- Choosing sustainable changes
- Avoiding extreme restriction
- Planning for hunger and cravings
- Accepting slower progress
- Building habits gradually

It also means:

- Being patient
- Being consistent
- Being realistic

These may not sound exciting, but they are effective.

Looking Ahead

Now that you understand why weight loss is difficult, the next step is to focus on something very practical:

How to approach eating in a realistic, sustainable way that supports long-term success.

In the next chapter, we will talk about diet, not as a short-term plan, but as a long-term strategy.

Main Points to Remember

- The body resists weight loss through biological mechanisms
- Hunger often increases after weight loss begins
- Metabolism may slow down
- Plateaus are common and expected
- The brain's reward system makes certain foods hard to resist
- Emotional eating patterns can return under stress
- Mental fatigue can affect consistency
- Unrealistic expectations lead to discouragement
- Small setbacks are normal and manageable
- Weight loss requires a long-term, realistic approach

What You Can Do Now

1. Adjust your expectations

Understand that:

- Progress may be slow
- Plateaus will happen

2. Prepare for hunger

Plan:

- Balanced meals
- Adequate protein and fiber

3. Accept imperfection

When small slips happen:

- Do not give up
- Return to your routine

4. Focus on consistency

Daily habits matter more than occasional perfection.

5. Be patient with yourself

This is a long-term process.

Chapter 5

Diet and Eating Patterns: A Practical, Sustainable Approach

When people think about weight loss, the first word that usually comes to mind is "diet."

And with that word often comes a sense of confusion.

Patients tell me:

"Doctor, there are so many diets. Which one is best?"

"Should I stop carbohydrates?"

"Should I try fasting?"

"Should I avoid fats?"

These are reasonable questions.

But over time, I have learned that focusing too much on finding the "perfect diet" often leads people in the wrong direction.

Because the truth is simple.

There is no single perfect diet for everyone.

What matters far more is whether your way of eating is something you can follow comfortably, consistently, and for a long time.

Why Most Diets Fail

Many diets fail not because they are completely wrong, but because they are difficult to sustain.

Some are:

- Too restrictive
- Too complicated
- Too different from a person's usual lifestyle
- Too focused on quick results

At the beginning, motivation is high. People follow the plan strictly. They may see early results.

But over time:

- Hunger increases
- Cravings return
- Social situations become difficult
- The plan feels tiring

Eventually, the person goes back to old eating patterns.

And the weight returns.

This cycle repeats so often that many people begin to feel that nothing will ever work.

But the real issue is not that change is impossible.

The issue is that the approach was not sustainable.

A Better Way to Think About Eating

Instead of asking,

"What diet should I follow?"

A more useful question is:

"What kind of eating pattern can I maintain for years?"

This shift is powerful.

Because long-term success depends not on short bursts of effort, but on steady, repeatable habits.

The Goal Is Not Perfection

You do not need to eat perfectly.

You need to eat **consistently better**.

That means:-

- Making reasonable choices most of the time
- Allowing flexibility when needed
- Avoiding extreme restriction

Perfection often leads to frustration.

Consistency leads to progress.

The Basics of a Balanced Plate

Rather than focusing on complicated rules, start with a simple structure.

A balanced meal generally includes:

1. Protein

Examples:

- Eggs
- Fish
- Chicken
- Beans
- Lentils
- Yogurt

Protein helps:

- Reduce hunger
- Maintain muscle
- Improve satiety

2. Fiber-Rich Foods

Examples:

- Vegetables

- Fruits
- Whole grains

Fiber helps:

- Improve digestion
- Increase fullness
- Stabilize blood sugar

3. Healthy Fats (in moderation)

Examples:

- Nuts
- Seeds
- Olive oil

Fats add flavor and satisfaction, but portion control is important.

Portion Awareness Matters More Than You Think

Many people eat healthy foods but still struggle with weight.

One common reason is portion size.

Even healthy foods, when eaten in large amounts, can lead to excess calorie intake.

You do not need to measure everything precisely.

But you do need awareness.

Simple strategies:

- Use smaller plates
- Avoid eating directly from large containers
- Pause before taking a second serving

The Problem with Sugary and Processed Foods

Highly processed foods are designed to be appealing.

They are:

- Easy to eat
- Highly palatable
- Often low in satiety

These foods do not make you feel full for long, and they often lead to overeating.

Reducing these foods can have a significant impact.

This does not mean you must eliminate them completely.

But reducing frequency and portion is very helpful.

Eating Patterns That Help

Certain patterns can support better control.

Regular Meal Timing

Eating at consistent times can help regulate hunger.

Skipping meals may lead to overeating later.

Mindful Eating

Pay attention to:

- What you are eating
- How much you are eating
- How you feel while eating

Avoid:

- Eating while distracted
- Eating too quickly

Reducing Late-Night Eating

Late-night eating often adds unnecessary calories.

It is usually driven by habit or emotion rather than hunger.

What About Popular Diets?

You may hear about:

- Low-carbohydrate diets
- Low-fat diets
- Intermittent fasting
- Keto diets

Some people do well on these approaches.

But the key question is not whether they work for someone

else.

The key question is:

Can you follow this comfortably over time?

If the answer is no, the results are unlikely to last.

Emotional Eating and Awareness

Many people eat for reasons beyond hunger.

They eat when they are:

- Stressed
- Bored
- Lonely
- Tired

Recognizing this is important.

Before eating, it can help to pause and ask:

"Am I truly hungry, or am I responding to something else?"

This simple question can change behavior over time.

Do Not Try to Change Everything at Once

One of the most common mistakes is trying to completely change eating habits overnight.

This often leads to failure.

Instead:

- Choose one or two changes
- Practice them consistently
- Add more changes gradually

For example:

- Replace sugary drinks
- Increase vegetables
- Reduce snacking

Small steps are more powerful than sudden, extreme changes.

Consistency Over Intensity

A plan followed at 70 percent consistency for months is far more effective than a perfect plan followed for two weeks.

This is one of the most important principles in weight management.

Do not aim to be perfect.

Aim to be consistent.

A Flexible Approach Works Best

Life includes:

- Family gatherings
- Social events

- Travel
- Occasional indulgence

A rigid plan often breaks under real-life conditions.

A flexible plan allows:

- Occasional variation
- Return to routine without guilt

This is how long-term success is built.

Looking Ahead

Now that we have discussed how to approach eating in a practical way, the next step is equally important.

How do we change behavior and habits in a lasting way?

In the next chapter, we will focus on behavior change, one of the most powerful tools for long-term success.

Main Points to Remember

- There is no single perfect diet for everyone
- Sustainability matters more than short-term results
- Balanced meals with protein, fiber, and healthy fats are helpful
- Portion awareness is essential

- Reducing processed and sugary foods can improve results
- Regular meal patterns support better control
- Emotional eating plays an important role
- Small, gradual changes are more effective than extreme changes
- Consistency is more important than perfection
- Flexibility supports long-term success

What You Can Do Now

1. Review your current eating habits

Ask yourself:

- Where can I improve?

2. Choose one change

For example:

- Reduce sugary drinks
- Add vegetables to meals

3. Practice mindful eating

Pay attention to:

- Hunger
- Portion size

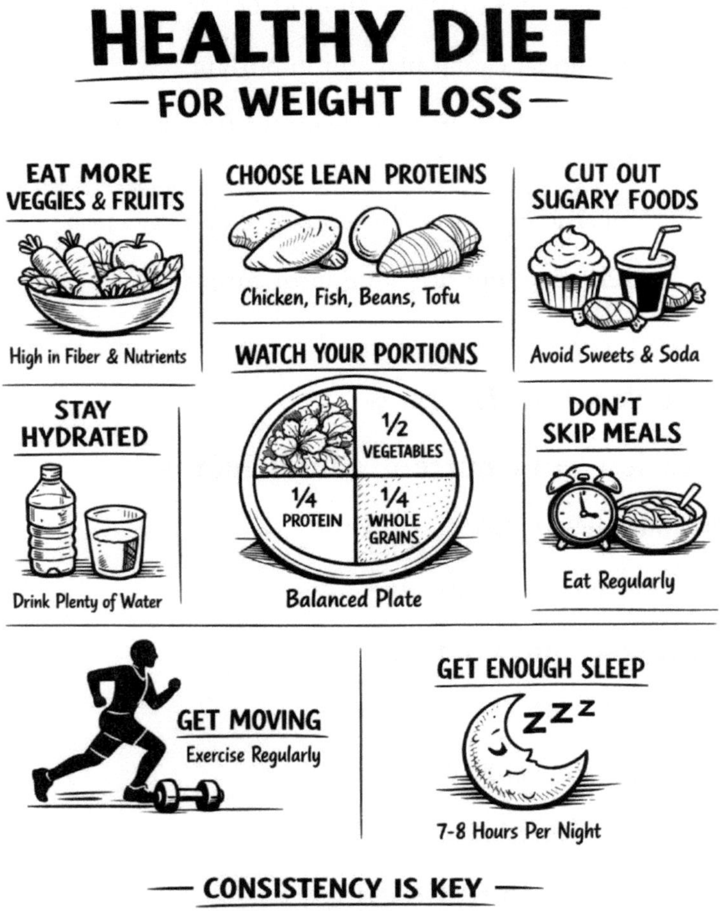
HEALTHY DIET
FOR WEIGHT LOSS
EAT MORE VEGGIES & FRUITS
High in Fiber & Nutrients
CHOOSE LEAN PROTEINS
Chicken, Fish, Beans, Tofu
CUT OUT SUGARY FOODS
Avoid Sweets & Soda
WATCH YOUR PORTIONS
1/2 VEGETABLES
1/4 PROTEIN
1/4 WHOLE GRAINS
Balanced Plate
STAY HYDRATED
Drink Plenty of Water
DON'T SKIP MEALS
Eat Regularly
GET MOVING
Exercise Regularly
GET ENOUGH SLEEP
7-8 Hours Per Night
CONSISTENCY IS KEY

4. Reduce one high-calorie habit

Identify:

- A snack
- A drink
- A routine

5. Stay consistent

Focus on:

- Small improvements
- Daily effort

Chapter 6

Behavior Change and Habit Formation

By this point, you already understand many important things.

You know what obesity is.

You know how it develops.

You understand why weight loss is difficult.

You have learned how to approach eating in a more practical way.

And yet, a very important question remains:

If I know what to do, why is it still so hard to do it consistently?

This is where behavior and habits come in.

Because in real life, success does not depend only on knowledge.

It depends on what you do every day.

Knowledge Is Not Enough

Many people know what healthy eating looks like.

They know:

- Vegetables are good
- Sugary drinks are not
- Portion control matters
- Physical activity helps

But knowing and doing are not the same.

A person may understand everything clearly, and still struggle to follow through.

This is not a failure of intelligence.

It is a challenge of behavior.

What Is a Habit?

A habit is something you do repeatedly, often without thinking.

For example:

- Having tea or coffee at a certain time
- Eating snacks while watching television
- Reaching for food when stressed

- Skipping activity after a long day

These actions become automatic over time.

You do not stop and decide each time. You simply do them.

This is why habits are powerful.

They reduce effort.

But they can work for you or against you.

How Habits Are Formed

Most habits follow a simple pattern:

Trigger '! Action '! Reward

- A trigger is something that starts the behavior
- The action is what you do
- The reward is what you get from it

For example:

- Trigger: Feeling stressed
- Action: Eating something sweet
- Reward: Temporary comfort

Over time, the brain begins to link the trigger with the action.

The pattern becomes automatic.

Why Old Habits Are Hard to Change

Habits are deeply ingrained.

Even when you try to change, old patterns remain in the background.

This is why:

- You may eat without thinking
- You may return to old routines during stress
- You may repeat behaviors you had planned to avoid

Changing habits requires more than willpower.

It requires awareness and strategy.

Start with Awareness

The first step in changing behavior is noticing it.

Many people eat automatically, without awareness.

Try to observe:

- When you eat
- What triggers your eating
- How you feel before and after

You may begin to see patterns.

For example:

- Eating late at night out of habit

- Snacking during stress
- Eating when bored

Awareness is the foundation of change.

Change One Habit at a Time

A common mistake is trying to change everything at once.

This often leads to frustration and failure.

Instead:

- Choose one habit
- Focus on it
- Practice consistently

For example:

- Reduce late-night snacking
- Avoid sugary drinks
- Add a short daily walk

Once one habit becomes stable, you can add another.

Replace, Do Not Just Remove

It is often easier to replace a habit than to eliminate it.

For example:

- Replace sugary drinks with water or unsweetened tea

- Replace evening snacking with a short walk
- Replace stress eating with a brief pause or relaxation

If you only remove a habit, the space it leaves behind often gets filled again.

Replacement works better.

Make It Easier to Succeed

Your environment plays a powerful role.

Small changes can make a big difference.

For example:

- Keep healthy foods easily available
- Avoid storing tempting foods in visible places
- Plan meals in advance
- Keep comfortable shoes ready for walking

When healthy choices are easier, you are more likely to follow them.

Plan for Difficult Moments

Behavior often breaks down during:

- Stress
- Fatigue
- Social situations

- Busy schedules

Instead of waiting for these moments, prepare for them.

Ask yourself:

"What will I do when I feel stressed?"

"What will I do when I am tired?"

Having a plan reduces impulsive decisions.

Do Not Aim for Perfection

Perfection is not required.

In fact, trying to be perfect often leads to failure.

There will be:

- Days when you do well
- Days when you do less well

What matters is returning to your routine.

A single mistake does not undo your progress.

Track Your Progress

Tracking helps build awareness and accountability.

This can be simple.

You may:

- Write down what you eat

- Track your steps
- Note your habits

This is not about judgment.

It is about understanding patterns.

Build Consistency, Not Intensity

Short bursts of intense effort are not sustainable.

Consistency matters more.

A small habit done daily is more powerful than a large effort done occasionally.

For example:

- Walking 20 minutes daily is better than exercising intensely once a week

Consistency builds momentum.

Be Patient with Change

Habits take time to change.

There will be:

- Slow progress
- Occasional setbacks

This is normal.

Behavior change is a gradual process.

Patience is essential.

The Role of Self-Compassion

Many people are very hard on themselves.

They think:

"I should have done better."

"I have no discipline."

This kind of thinking often makes things worse.

A more helpful approach is:

- Acknowledge the difficulty
- Learn from mistakes
- Continue moving forward

Self-compassion is not weakness.

It supports persistence.

You Are Rewiring Patterns

When you change habits, you are not just changing behavior.

You are changing patterns that may have been present for years.

This takes time.

But with repetition, new patterns become easier.

What once felt difficult becomes more natural.

Looking Ahead

Now that you understand how behavior and habits work, we are ready to explore another important dimension:

The role of psychological and emotional factors in weight gain and weight loss.

In the next chapter, we will look deeper into emotions, mindset, and their impact on eating and weight.

Main Points to Remember

- Knowledge alone is not enough for weight loss
- Habits drive daily behavior
- Habits follow a pattern: trigger, action, reward
- Old habits are difficult to change but can be modified
- Awareness is the first step
- Change one habit at a time
- Replacing habits works better than removing them
- Environment influences behavior
- Consistency is more important than intensity
- Self-compassion supports long-term success

What You Can Do Now

1. Identify one habit

Behavior Changes for Weight Loss

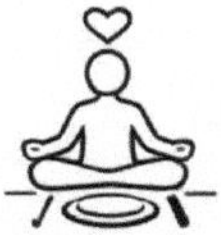

Mindful Eating

Eat Slowly, Avoid Distractions

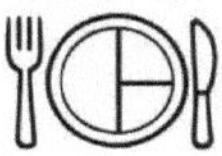

Portion Control

Watch Your Serving Sizes

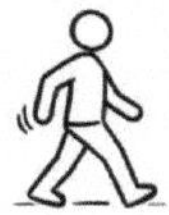

Regular Activity

Exercise Daily

Healthy Food Choices

Choose Nutritious Foods

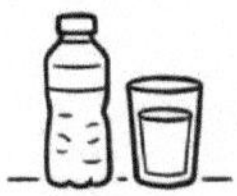

Hydration

Drink Plenty of Water

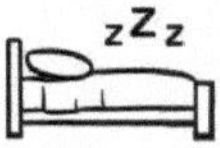

Sleep

Get 7-8 Hours Per Night

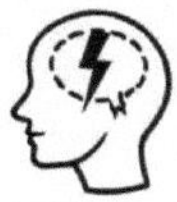

Stress Control

Manage Your Stress

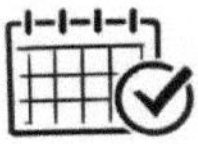

Consistency

Stick to Your Plan

Choose something specific:

- Late-night eating
- Sugary drinks
- Sedentary routine

2. Understand the trigger

Ask:

- When does this happen?
- Why does it happen?

3. Plan a replacement

Decide:

- What will I do instead?

4. Track your progress

Keep it simple:

- Daily check

5. Stay consistent

Focus on:

- Small daily improvement

Chapter 7
Psychological Factors and Emotional Eating

By now, you understand that weight is not only about food and activity.

There is another layer that is often less visible, but just as powerful.

It is the emotional side of eating.

Many people tell me, sometimes after a long pause,

"Doctor, I don't think I eat only because I am hungry."

That realization is very important.

Because for many individuals, eating is closely connected to emotions, thoughts, and daily experiences.

Eating Is Not Always About Hunger

In an ideal situation, we eat when we are physically hungry and stop when we feel satisfied.

But in real life, eating is often influenced by many other factors.

People eat when they are:

- Stressed
- Tired
- Bored
- Lonely
- Celebrating
- Rewarding themselves

Food becomes more than nutrition. It becomes comfort, distraction, reward, and sometimes even habit.

This is completely human.

But when this pattern becomes frequent, it can contribute to weight gain.

Understanding Emotional Eating

Emotional eating happens when food is used to cope with feelings rather than hunger.

For example:

- After a stressful day, you may reach for something sweet

- During loneliness, eating may feel comforting
- When bored, food may provide stimulation

The relief is usually temporary.

Afterward, there may be:

- Guilt
- Frustration
- Disappointment

And this can create a cycle that repeats over time.

The Emotional Eating Cycle

Many people find themselves in a pattern like this:

- Emotional discomfort
- Eating for relief
- Temporary comfort
- Guilt or regret
- Increased emotional distress
- Return to eating

This cycle can be difficult to break.

Not because a person lacks discipline, but because the pattern is deeply learned.

Stress and Its Impact

Stress is one of the most powerful triggers for emotional eating.

When you are under stress:

- Your body produces stress hormones
- Cravings for high-calorie foods increase
- Self-control may decrease

At the same time, stress often reduces energy and motivation.

This combination makes it easier to overeat and harder to stay consistent.

The Role of Mood

Mood also influences eating behavior.

Some people notice:

- Eating more when they feel low
- Using food as a way to feel better
- Turning to familiar foods for comfort

This does not mean something is wrong with you.

It means your mind has learned to associate food with emotional relief.

The Role of Habit in Emotional Eating

Over time, emotional eating can become a habit.

It may begin as an occasional response to stress or boredom. But with repetition, it becomes automatic.

For example:

- Feeling stressed may immediately lead to eating
- Watching television may automatically include snacking
- Finishing a meal may create a habit of having something sweet

At that point, the behavior may happen even without strong emotion.

This is where emotional eating and habit begin to overlap.

Understanding this helps you approach the problem more calmly and more effectively.

Learning to Pause

One of the most powerful skills you can develop is the ability to pause.

Before eating, take a moment and ask yourself:

"Am I physically hungry, or am I responding to something else?"

This simple question creates awareness.

You may not always change your behavior immediately, but you begin to notice it.

And awareness is the first step toward change.

Recognizing Your Triggers

Each person has their own triggers.

Common triggers include:

- Stress from work or family
- Loneliness or isolation
- Boredom during quiet moments
- Fatigue at the end of the day
- Certain environments or routines

Try to observe patterns.

When do you tend to eat without hunger?

What situations lead to overeating?

When you recognize your triggers, you can begin to prepare for them.

Finding Alternatives to Emotional Eating

Food is one way to cope with emotions, but it is not the only way.

It helps to develop alternative responses.

For example:

- Take a short walk
- Step outside for fresh air
- Call a friend or family member

- Sit quietly and take a few slow breaths
- Engage in a simple activity like reading or listening to music

These alternatives may not feel as immediately satisfying as food.

But over time, they can become new, healthier patterns.

Managing Stress in a Healthier Way

Since stress is such a common trigger, learning to manage it is important.

This does not require complicated techniques.

Simple practices can help:

- Taking short breaks during the day
- Getting regular sleep
- Spending a few minutes in quiet reflection
- Engaging in light physical activity

These small steps reduce emotional pressure and make overeating less likely.

Do Not Fight Every Emotion with Food

It is natural to want to avoid discomfort.

But not every emotion needs to be "fixed" immediately.

Sometimes it is enough to:

- Notice the feeling
- Allow it to pass
- Avoid reacting impulsively

Emotions often rise and fall.

If you can give them a little time, the urge to eat may pass as well.

Reducing Guilt and Self-Criticism

Many people are very harsh with themselves after emotional eating.

They think:

"I should have controlled myself."

"I have no discipline."

This kind of thinking often makes things worse.

It increases stress and makes the cycle stronger.

A better approach is:

- Acknowledge what happened
- Understand why it happened
- Move forward without harsh judgment

You are learning, not failing.

Building Emotional Awareness

Emotional awareness means recognizing what you feel and how it affects your behavior.

Ask yourself:

- What am I feeling right now?
- What do I really need at this moment?

Sometimes, the need is not food.

It may be:

- Rest
- Support
- Distraction
- Relaxation

Learning to recognize this can change your response.

Progress, Not Perfection

Emotional eating will not disappear overnight.

There will still be moments when you eat for reasons other than hunger.

That is normal.

What matters is:

- Increasing awareness
- Reducing frequency

- Improving your response over time

Small improvements lead to meaningful change.

A More Compassionate Approach

One of the most important shifts is moving from self-criticism to self-understanding.

You are not dealing with a simple problem.

You are dealing with patterns built over years, influenced by life experiences, emotions, and habits.

Change takes time.

And it requires patience.

Looking Ahead

Now that we have explored the emotional and psychological side of eating, we move to another essential part of weight management:

Physical activity and exercise, how they help, and how to make them part of your daily life in a realistic way.

Main Points to Remember

- Eating is often influenced by emotions, not just hunger
- Emotional eating is common and understandable

- Stress, mood, and habits all play a role
- Emotional eating often follows a repeating cycle
- Awareness is the first step to change
- Pausing before eating can help you make better decisions
- Identifying triggers allows better preparation
- Alternative coping strategies can reduce reliance on food
- Self-compassion is more helpful than self-criticism
- Progress comes gradually over time

What You Can Do Now

1. Observe your patterns

For a few days, notice:

- When you eat without hunger
- What you are feeling at that time

2. Practice the pause

Before eating, ask:

- Am I truly hungry?

3. Identify one trigger

Choose one common situation:

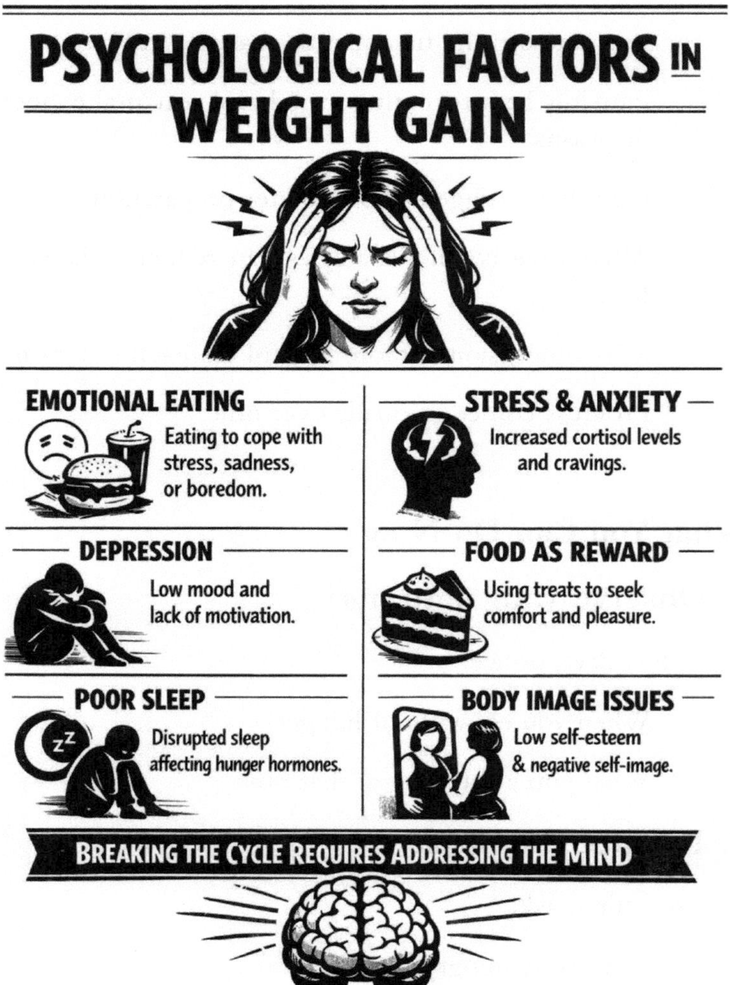
PSYCHOLOGICAL FACTORS IN WEIGHT GAIN
EMOTIONAL EATING
Eating to cope with stress, sadness, or boredom.
STRESS & ANXIETY
Increased cortisol levels and cravings.
DEPRESSION
Low mood and lack of motivation.
FOOD AS REWARD
Using treats to seek comfort and pleasure.
POOR SLEEP
Disrupted sleep affecting hunger hormones.
BODY IMAGE ISSUES
Low self-esteem & negative self-image.
BREAKING THE CYCLE REQUIRES ADDRESSING THE MIND

- Stress
- Boredom
- Evening routine

4. Plan an alternative

Decide in advance:

- What will I do instead of eating?

5. Be kind to yourself

When mistakes happen:

- Learn from them and move forward

Chapter 8

Physical Activity and Exercise: A Realistic Approach

When people think about weight loss, they often feel that exercise must play a major role.

At the same time, many feel uncertain.

Patients tell me:

"Doctor, I don't have time to exercise."

"I feel too tired after work."

"I am not able to go to the gym."

"Will walking even help?"

These are very common concerns.

Let me reassure you at the beginning:

You do not need extreme exercise to improve your health or support weight loss.

What you need is **regular, realistic movement that fits your life**.

Why Physical Activity Matters

Physical activity supports weight management in several important ways.

It helps:

- Burn calories
- Maintain muscle mass
- Improve metabolism
- Reduce stress
- Improve sleep
- Increase energy

Even beyond weight, activity improves overall health.

It supports:

- Heart health
- Blood sugar control
- Joint mobility
- Mental well-being

So while diet plays a major role in weight loss, physical activity plays a major role in **long-term success and overall health**.

Exercise Is Not Just About the Gym

Many people think exercise means:

- Going to the gym
- Lifting heavy weights
- Running long distances

This is not necessary.

Physical activity includes:

- Walking
- Climbing stairs
- Household work
- Gardening
- Light stretching

Movement throughout the day matters.

In fact, regular daily movement can be more sustainable than occasional intense workouts.

Start Where You Are

You do not need to begin at a high level.

Start with your current ability.

If you are not active:

- Begin with short walks

- Even 10 to 15 minutes is useful

If you already walk:

- Increase duration gradually
- Add a little pace

The goal is not to do everything at once.

The goal is to begin.

Walking: A Simple and Powerful Tool

Walking is one of the most practical forms of exercise.

It requires:

- No special equipment
- No training
- No gym membership

Benefits of walking:

- Easy to start
- Low risk of injury
- Can be done almost anywhere
- Can be adjusted to your level

Try to build toward:

- 30 minutes most days of the week

This can be done all at once or in shorter sessions.

Consistency Matters More Than Intensity

A common mistake is doing too much too soon.

This often leads to:

- Fatigue
- Soreness
- Loss of motivation

Instead:

- Focus on regular activity
- Keep it manageable

A moderate routine followed consistently is far more effective than intense effort that cannot be sustained.

Strength Matters Too

As we age, we tend to lose muscle.

Muscle is important because it:

- Supports metabolism
- Improves strength
- Helps with daily activities

Simple strength exercises can help:

- Light weights
- Resistance bands

- Bodyweight exercises

You do not need complex routines.

Even basic strengthening, done a few times a week, can be beneficial.

Reduce Sitting Time

Many people sit for long hours.

Even if you exercise once a day, long periods of sitting can still affect health.

Try to:

- Stand up every hour
- Walk for a few minutes
- Stretch briefly

These small movements add up.

Make Activity Part of Your Routine

Activity is easier when it becomes part of your day.

For example:

- Walk after meals
- Take stairs when possible
- Park a little farther away
- Schedule a daily walk

When activity is built into your routine, it requires less effort to maintain.

Overcoming Common Barriers

"I Don't Have Time"

Start small:

- 10 to 15 minutes
- Build gradually

"I Feel Too Tired"

Paradoxically, regular activity often increases energy over time.

"I Am Not Fit Enough"

You do not need to be fit to start.

You become fit by starting.

"I Cannot Go to the Gym"

You do not need a gym.

Your body and a small space are enough.

Listen to Your Body

Activity should be safe and comfortable.

- Start slowly
- Increase gradually

- Avoid pushing through pain

If you have medical conditions, consult your doctor before starting a new routine.

Activity and Weight Loss Expectations

Exercise alone may not lead to large weight loss.

But it plays a key role in:

- Maintaining weight loss
- Improving body composition
- Supporting long-term success

Think of activity as a partner to diet, not a replacement.

Enjoyment Makes It Sustainable

You are more likely to continue what you enjoy.

Choose activities you like:

- Walking outdoors
- Light sports
- Dancing
- Group activities

Enjoyment increases consistency.

A Long-Term View

Physical activity is not a short-term effort.

It is part of a healthy lifestyle.

Over time, regular movement becomes:

- Easier
- More natural
- More rewarding

This is where real benefit lies.

Looking Ahead

Now that we have covered diet, behavior, emotions, and activity, we move to the next important area:

Medical treatments, when they are needed, and how they can support weight loss.

Main Points to Remember

- Physical activity supports weight loss and overall health
- Exercise does not need to be intense to be effective
- Walking is a simple and powerful option
- Consistency is more important than intensity
- Strength training helps maintain muscle

- Reducing sitting time is important
- Activity should fit your daily routine
- Barriers can be managed with small steps
- Exercise supports long-term weight control
- Enjoyable activities are easier to sustain

What You Can Do Now

1. Start small

Begin with:

- 10 to 15 minutes of walking

2. Build gradually

Increase:

- Time
- Frequency

3. Reduce sitting

Stand and move:

- Every hour

4. Add simple strength activity

Try:

- Light resistance exercises

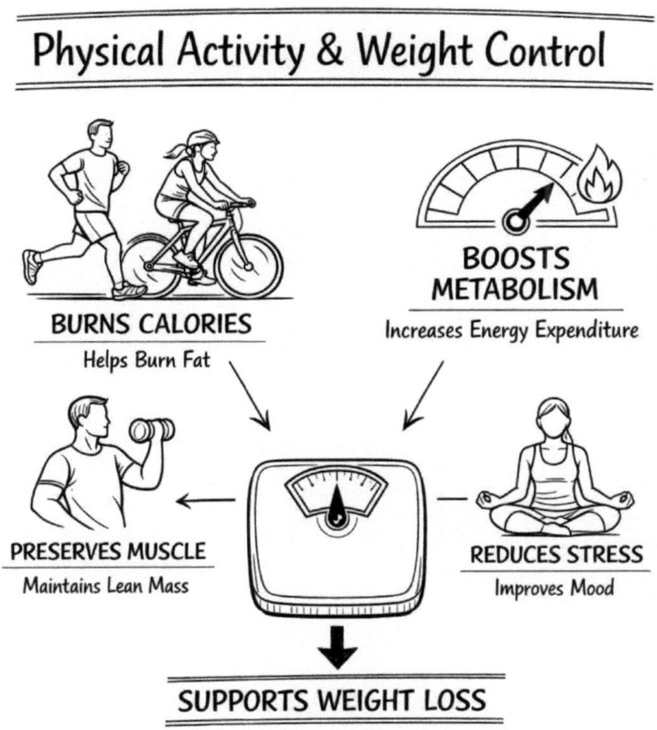
Physical Activity & Weight Control
BURNS CALORIES
Helps Burn Fat
BOOSTS METABOLISM
Increases Energy Expenditure
PRESERVES MUSCLE
Maintains Lean Mass
REDUCES STRESS
Improves Mood
SUPPORTS WEIGHT LOSS

5. Stay consistent

Focus on:

- Daily movement

Chapter 9
When Is Medical Treatment Needed?

Up to this point, we have focused on lifestyle changes.

We discussed:

- Eating patterns
- Behavior and habits
- Emotional factors
- Physical activity

These form the foundation of weight management.

But an important question often comes up at this stage:

"Doctor, what if I have tried all this and still cannot lose enough weight?"

This is a very reasonable question.

Because for some individuals, lifestyle changes alone may not be enough.

Understanding the Limits of Lifestyle Alone

Lifestyle changes are essential.

They improve health, build better habits, and form the base of any long-term plan.

But in some cases:

- Weight loss is limited
- Progress is slow or inconsistent
- Weight regain occurs despite effort

This does not mean the person has failed.

It may reflect the biology of obesity.

As we discussed earlier:

- The body resists weight loss
- Hunger increases
- Metabolism adapts

In some individuals, these factors are strong enough that additional help is needed.

When Should Medical Treatment Be Considered?

Medical treatment may be considered when:

- **Body Mass Index (BMI) is 30 or higher**, or
- **BMI is 27 or higher with related health conditions**, such as:

o Diabetes

o High blood pressure

o Sleep apnea

o High cholesterol

It may also be appropriate when:

- Lifestyle efforts have been consistent but insufficient
- Weight is affecting health or quality of life
- There is a high risk of future complications

This decision is always individualized.

Obesity as a Medical Condition

One of the most important shifts in recent years is recognizing obesity as a **chronic medical condition**.

This means:

- It develops over time
- It tends to persist
- It often requires long-term management

This is similar to conditions like:

- High blood pressure

- Diabetes

We do not expect those conditions to improve with willpower alone.

In the same way, some individuals may need medical support for weight management.

Types of Medical Treatment

Medical treatment for weight loss generally falls into three categories:

1. Medications

These help by:

- Reducing appetite
- Increasing fullness
- Improving metabolic control

We will discuss these in detail in the next chapters.

2. Advanced Medical Therapies (Including GLP-1)

These are newer treatments that:

- Act on appetite regulation
- Improve metabolic function

They have shown significant results in many patients.

We will explore them carefully and in detail.

3. Surgical Options

For some individuals, surgery may be considered.

These procedures:

- Reduce stomach size
- Alter digestive processes

They can lead to significant weight loss and health improvement.

We will discuss this in a later chapter.

Medical Treatment Is Not a Shortcut

One common concern is:

"Is taking medication an easy way out?"

The answer is no.

Medical treatment is not a replacement for lifestyle change.

It is a support.

Even with medication:

- Healthy eating is still important
- Physical activity remains necessary
- Behavior change is essential

Think of medical treatment as an additional tool, not a substitute.

Choosing the Right Approach

Not everyone needs medical treatment.

And not every treatment is suitable for everyone.

The right approach depends on:

- Your health condition
- Your weight history
- Your response to lifestyle changes
- Your preferences and goals

This is why individual assessment is important.

Safety and Supervision

Medical treatments should always be used under proper guidance.

This helps:

- Ensure safety
- Monitor progress
- Adjust treatment when needed

Self-prescribing or using unverified products can be harmful.

It is important to rely on evidence-based treatments.

Setting Realistic Expectations

Medical treatments can help.

But they are not magic.

Results may include:

- Moderate to significant weight loss
- Improved control over appetite
- Better metabolic health

But:

- Effort is still required
- Results take time
- Not everyone responds the same way

Understanding this helps avoid disappointment.

The Importance of a Combined Approach

The most effective strategy combines:

- Lifestyle changes
- Behavioral adjustments
- Medical support when needed

This integrated approach leads to better and more sustainable outcomes.

A Balanced Perspective

Medical treatment should not be viewed as:

- A failure
- A weakness
- A last resort

It is simply one part of modern medical care.

For some people, it can make a significant difference.

For others, it may not be necessary.

The key is to make an informed decision.

Looking Ahead

In the next chapter, we will explore:

Weight loss medications, how they work, their benefits, risks, and what you should realistically expect.

Main Points to Remember

- Lifestyle changes are essential but may not always be enough
- Obesity is a chronic medical condition
- Medical treatment may be considered based on BMI and health conditions
- Treatment options include medications, advanced

therapies, and surgery

- Medical treatment is a support, not a shortcut
- Individualized care is important
- Medical supervision ensures safety
- Realistic expectations are essential
- Combining approaches leads to better results

What You Can Do Now

1. Reflect on your progress

Ask yourself:

- Have I tried lifestyle changes consistently?
- What results have I seen?

2. Assess your health

Consider:

- Do I have weight-related health conditions?

3. Stay open to options

Understand that:

- Medical support may be appropriate in some cases

4. Prepare for discussion

If needed, talk with your doctor about:

- Available options

- Benefits and risks

5. Focus on long-term success

Think beyond short-term results.

Chapter 10

Weight Loss Medications: What You Should Know

At some point in the journey, many patients ask me a direct question:

"Doctor, are there medicines that can help me lose weight?"

Sometimes the question is asked with hope.

Sometimes with hesitation.

And sometimes with concern.

People wonder:

"Are these medicines safe?"

"Do they really work?"

"Will I become dependent on them?"

These are important and thoughtful questions.

In this chapter, let us look at weight loss medications in a clear and balanced way.

Why Consider Medication at All?

As we discussed earlier, weight loss is not always easy.

Even with sincere effort:

- Hunger may increase
- Cravings may persist
- Progress may slow

For some individuals, these challenges are strong enough that lifestyle changes alone do not lead to sufficient results.

In such cases, medication may help.

The purpose of medication is not to replace effort.

It is to **support your efforts**.

How Do Weight Loss Medications Work?

Different medications work in different ways.

Most commonly, they help by:

Reducing Appetite

They act on the brain to decrease hunger signals.

Increasing Fullness

You may feel satisfied with smaller portions.

Slowing Digestion

Food remains in the stomach longer, helping you feel full.

Affecting Food Absorption

Some medications reduce how much fat is absorbed from food.

These effects can make it easier to eat less without constant struggle.

What Kind of Results Can You Expect?

It is important to have realistic expectations.

Most weight loss medications lead to:

- **About 5 to 10 percent reduction in body weight**

Some people lose more. Some lose less.

The key point is this:

Even moderate weight loss can improve:

- Blood pressure
- Blood sugar
- Joint symptoms
- Overall health

Medication helps move you in the right direction.

Benefits Beyond the Scale

Weight loss medications may provide additional benefits.

These can include:

- Better control of appetite
- Reduced cravings
- Improved metabolic health
- Support for long-term weight management

For some individuals, this makes a meaningful difference.

Possible Side Effects

All medications can have side effects.

Common side effects may include:

- Nausea
- Constipation or diarrhea
- Headache
- Dry mouth

These are often mild and may improve over time.

However, side effects vary depending on the medication and the individual.

This is why monitoring is important.

Safety and Individual Suitability

Not every medication is suitable for everyone.

Factors to consider include:

- Medical history
- Current medications
- Existing health conditions

Some medications may not be appropriate for people with:

- Certain heart conditions
- Uncontrolled high blood pressure
- Specific psychiatric conditions

This is why medical evaluation is essential.

Medical Supervision Is Important

Weight loss medications should always be used under medical guidance.

This helps to:

- Choose the right medication
- Monitor progress
- Adjust treatment if needed
- Identify side effects early

Using medications without proper supervision can be unsafe.

Medications Are Not a Cure

It is very important to understand this clearly.

Medications do not cure obesity.

They help manage it.

If lifestyle habits are not maintained:

- Benefits may be limited
- Weight may return

The best results come when medication is combined with:

- Healthy eating
- Physical activity
- Behavior change

What Happens If You Stop the Medication?

This is a common concern.

In many cases:

- Appetite may increase again
- Weight regain may occur

This reflects the ongoing nature of weight regulation.

It does not mean the medication failed.

For some individuals, longer-term use may be needed.

Cost and Practical Considerations

Some medications can be expensive.

Insurance coverage varies.

This may influence the choice of treatment.

It is important to consider:

- Cost
- Access
- Long-term feasibility

A Balanced Perspective

Weight loss medications are neither a miracle nor something to avoid completely.

They are tools.

For the right person, used in the right way, they can be helpful.

For others, they may not be necessary.

The goal is not to use medication for everyone.

The goal is to use it wisely when appropriate.

Looking Ahead

In the next chapter, we will focus on one of the most important advances in recent years:

GLP-1 medications, how they work, why they are effective,

and what you should know before considering them.

Main Points to Remember

- Weight loss medications may be helpful for some individuals
- They support lifestyle changes, not replace them
- They work by reducing appetite, increasing fullness, or affecting digestion
- Typical weight loss is moderate but meaningful
- Side effects are possible and vary
- Medical supervision is essential
- Medications are not a cure for obesity
- Weight may return after stopping treatment
- Cost and access are important considerations
- They should be used as part of a comprehensive plan

What You Can Do Now

1. Reflect on your needs

Ask yourself:

- Have I struggled despite consistent effort?

2. Learn about options

Understand:

- Benefits
- Risks

3. Prepare for a discussion

If appropriate, talk to your doctor about:

- Suitability
- Expectations

4. Stay realistic

Remember:

- Medication supports effort
- It does not replace it

5. Focus on long-term success

Think beyond quick results.

Chapter 11

GLP-1 Medications: A New Era in Weight Loss

In recent years, one topic comes up again and again in my office.

"Doctor, I keep hearing about these new weight loss injections."

"Are they really effective?"

"Are they safe?"

There is a lot of interest, and also a lot of confusion.

Some people see them as a breakthrough.

Others are unsure or even skeptical.

Let us take a clear and balanced look.

What Are GLP-1 Medications?

GLP-1 stands for **glucagon-like peptide-1**.

It is a natural hormone already present in your body.

This hormone plays an important role in:

- Regulating appetite
- Controlling blood sugar
- Slowing stomach emptying

GLP-1 medications are designed to mimic this natural hormone.

They do not introduce something foreign.

They enhance a system your body already uses.

How Do They Work?

GLP-1 medications work in several helpful ways.

1. Reducing Hunger

They act on the brain to decrease appetite.

You feel less desire to eat.

2. Increasing Fullness

You feel satisfied sooner during meals.

Portion sizes naturally become smaller.

3. Slowing Digestion

Food stays in the stomach longer.

This prolongs the feeling of fullness.

4. Improving Blood Sugar Control

They help regulate insulin and glucose levels, especially useful for people with diabetes or insulin resistance.

Together, these effects make eating less feel more natural and less forced.

How Effective Are They?

GLP-1 medications are among the most effective medical treatments for weight loss available today.

Many individuals experience:

- Noticeable reduction in appetite
- Gradual, steady weight loss

In clinical studies and real-world experience:

- Weight loss may reach **10 to 15 percent or more of body weight**

However, results vary.

Some people lose more, some less.

Benefits Beyond Weight Loss

One of the most important advantages of GLP-1 medications is that their benefits go beyond weight reduction.

They may help:

- Improve blood sugar control
- Reduce the risk of diabetes
- Lower blood pressure
- Improve cardiovascular health in certain individuals

For many patients, these additional benefits are just as important as weight loss itself.

Common Side Effects

Like all medications, GLP-1 therapies can have side effects.

The most common include:

- Nausea
- Vomiting
- Diarrhea or constipation
- Reduced appetite

These are usually mild and tend to improve over time.

Starting at a low dose and gradually increasing helps reduce these effects.

Important Safety Considerations

GLP-1 medications are generally safe when used appropriately.

However, they are not suitable for everyone.

They may not be recommended for individuals with:

- Certain thyroid conditions
- Specific endocrine tumors
- Severe gastrointestinal disorders

Rare side effects can occur, so medical supervision is important.

How Are These Medications Taken?

Most GLP-1 medications are given as injections.

Depending on the type:

- Some are taken daily
- Others are taken once weekly

The injection is usually given under the skin.

Many patients feel hesitant at first, but most become comfortable quickly.

Cost and Access

One practical challenge is cost.

These medications can be expensive, and insurance coverage varies.

Access depends on:

- Insurance policies
- Medical eligibility
- Availability

This is an important part of the decision-making process.

What Happens If You Stop?

This is one of the most important questions.

When the medication is stopped:

- Appetite may increase again
- Weight regain can occur

This reflects the chronic nature of obesity.

It does not mean the treatment failed.

For many individuals, long-term use may be needed to maintain results.

Are GLP-1 Medications Right for You?

These medications can be very helpful for certain individuals, especially those who:

- Struggle with strong appetite or cravings
- Have obesity-related health conditions
- Have not achieved sufficient results with lifestyle

changes

However, they are not necessary for everyone.

The decision depends on:

- Individual health status
- Goals
- Preferences
- Medical guidance

A Balanced Perspective

It is easy to think of GLP-1 medications as a complete solution.

They are not.

They are a powerful tool, but still part of a larger plan.

Best results come when they are combined with:

- Healthy eating
- Regular physical activity
- Behavior change

Looking Ahead

In the next chapter, we will discuss another important option:

Weight loss surgery, when it is considered, how it works, and what to expect.

Main Points to Remember

- GLP-1 is a natural hormone involved in appetite and blood sugar regulation
- GLP-1 medications mimic this hormone
- They reduce hunger and increase fullness
- They are among the most effective weight loss medications available
- They offer benefits beyond weight loss
- Common side effects are usually mild
- They are not suitable for everyone
- Most are given as injections
- Weight may return after stopping
- They work best as part of a comprehensive plan

What You Can Do Now

1. Understand the option

Learn:

- How these medications work
- Their benefits and limitations

2. Reflect on your needs

Ask:

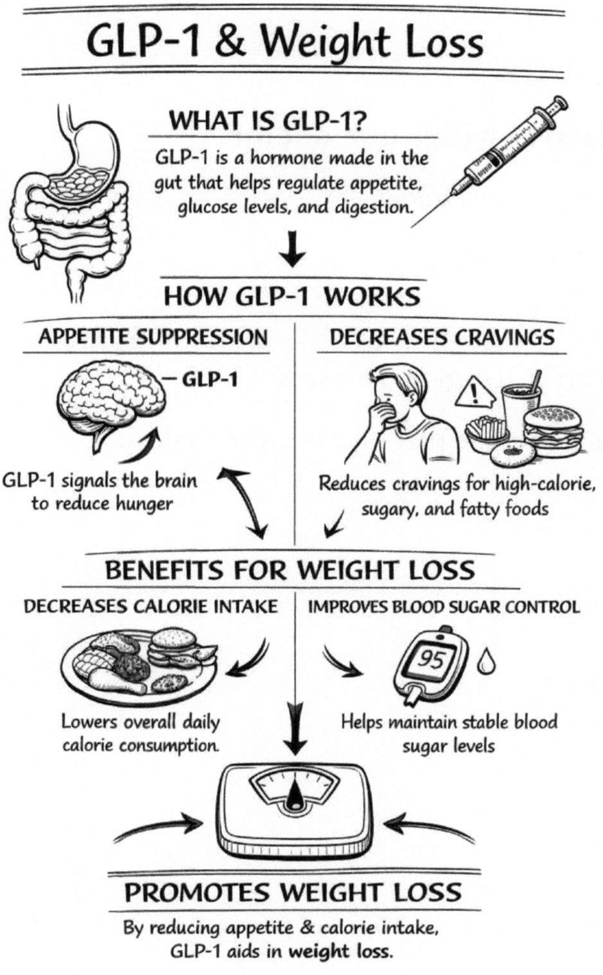
GLP-1 & Weight Loss
WHAT IS GLP-1?
GLP-1 is a hormone made in the gut that helps regulate appetite, glucose levels, and digestion.
HOW GLP-1 WORKS
APPETITE SUPPRESSION
— GLP-1
GLP-1 signals the brain to reduce hunger
DECREASES CRAVINGS
Reduces cravings for high-calorie, sugary, and fatty foods
BENEFITS FOR WEIGHT LOSS
DECREASES CALORIE INTAKE
Lowers overall daily calorie consumption
IMPROVES BLOOD SUGAR CONTROL
95
Helps maintain stable blood sugar levels
PROMOTES WEIGHT LOSS
By reducing appetite & calorie intake, GLP-1 aids in weight loss.

- Am I struggling with appetite control?

3. Consider practical factors

Think about:

- Cost
- Access

4. Discuss with your doctor

If interested, talk about:

- Suitability
- Risks

5. Keep a long-term view

Medication is one part of a broader strategy.

Chapter 12

Weight Loss Surgery: An Important Option for Some

When the topic of weight loss surgery comes up, people often have mixed feelings.

Some feel hopeful.

Some feel anxious.

Many are simply unsure.

Patients ask me:

"Doctor, is surgery my last option?"

"Is it safe?"

"Will it really help?"

These are thoughtful and very reasonable questions.

Weight loss surgery, also known as **bariatric surgery**, is not for everyone. But for certain individuals, it can be a very effective and life-changing treatment.

When Is Surgery Considered?

Surgery is usually considered in the following situations:

- **Body Mass Index (BMI) is 40 or higher**, or
- **BMI is 35 or higher with serious health conditions,** such as:

  o Diabetes

  o High blood pressure

  o Sleep apnea

It may also be considered when:

- Other methods have not produced sufficient results
- Weight is significantly affecting health and daily life

This decision is not based on weight alone. It involves a careful evaluation of overall health and readiness.

Common Types of Surgery

There are several types of bariatric surgery. The most commonly performed include:

1. Sleeve Gastrectomy (Gastric Sleeve)

A portion of the stomach is removed, leaving a smaller, tube-shaped stomach.

This leads to:

- Reduced food intake
- Reduced hunger

2. Gastric Bypass

The stomach is made smaller and connected directly to a lower part of the intestine.

This results in:

- Reduced food intake
- Changes in how nutrients are absorbed

Each procedure has its own benefits and risks. The choice depends on individual factors and medical advice.

How Surgery Helps

Weight loss surgery works in more than one way.

It:

- Limits how much you can eat
- Changes hunger-related hormones
- Alters how the body processes food

Many patients notice:

- Reduced appetite

- Feeling full sooner
- Less interest in large meals

These changes make weight loss more achievable.

Expected Results

Weight loss after surgery can be significant.

Many individuals lose:

- About **20 to 35 percent of their body weight**

In addition, many experience improvement in:

- Diabetes
- Blood pressure
- Sleep apnea
- Joint pain

For some, these improvements can be dramatic.

Benefits Beyond Weight Loss

Surgery can lead to important improvements in daily life.

Patients often report:

- Better energy
- Improved mobility
- Greater confidence

- Better quality of life

These changes can be just as meaningful as the weight loss itself.

Risks and Complications

As with any surgery, there are risks.

Short-term risks may include:

- Infection
- Bleeding
- Reactions to anesthesia

Long-term considerations may include:

- Nutritional deficiencies
- Digestive changes
- Need for lifelong supplementation

These risks are generally low when surgery is performed in experienced centers, but they must be understood.

Life After Surgery

Surgery is not the end of the journey.

It is the beginning of a new phase.

After surgery, patients need to:

- Follow specific dietary guidelines

- Eat smaller portions
- Take vitamin and mineral supplements
- Attend regular follow-up visits

Eating habits change significantly.

Meals become smaller, and eating slowly becomes important.

Over time, most people adjust well.

The Importance of Commitment

Surgery is a powerful tool, but not a cure.

Long-term success depends on:

- Healthy eating habits
- Regular physical activity
- Ongoing follow-up

Without these, weight regain can occur.

Commitment remains essential.

Emotional Adjustment

Weight loss after surgery can bring emotional changes.

Some people feel:

- Increased confidence
- Improved mood

Others may experience:

- Adjustment challenges
- Changes in relationships
- Concerns about body image

Support from family, healthcare providers, or counseling can be helpful.

Is Surgery the Right Choice for You?

Surgery may be appropriate if:

- Weight is significantly affecting health
- Other methods have not worked
- You are willing to commit to long-term changes

It is not the right choice for everyone.

A careful, informed discussion with your doctor is essential.

A Balanced View

Weight loss surgery should not be seen as:

- Something to fear unnecessarily
- Or something to choose lightly

It is a medical option with clear benefits and real responsibilities.

For the right person, it can be life-changing.

Looking Ahead

In the next chapter, we will focus on a very important topic:

How to prevent weight regain and maintain your progress over the long term.

Main Points to Remember

- Weight loss surgery is considered for individuals with higher BMI and related conditions
- Common procedures include gastric sleeve and gastric bypass
- Surgery works by reducing intake and altering hunger signals
- Significant weight loss and health improvement are possible
- Risks exist and should be understood
- Lifelong lifestyle changes and follow-up are required
- Surgery is a tool, not a cure
- Emotional adjustment may be needed
- The decision should be individualized

What You Can Do Now

1. Reflect on your situation

Ask yourself:

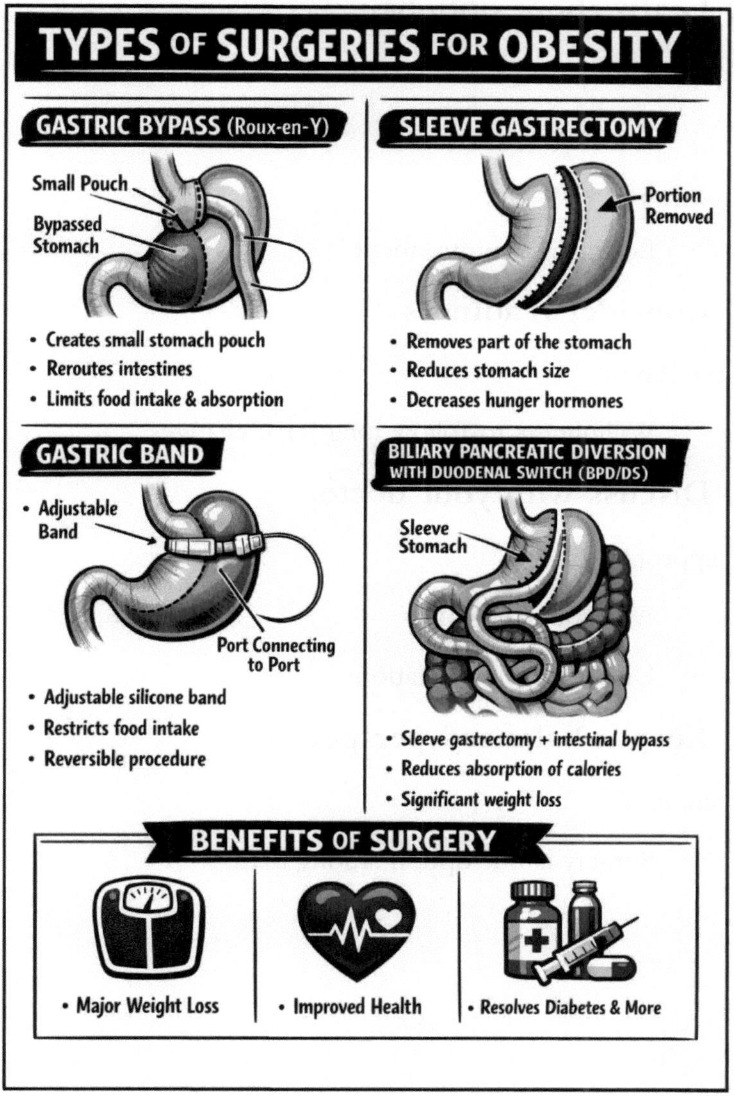
TYPES OF SURGERIES FOR OBESITY
GASTRIC BYPASS (Roux-en-Y)
Small Pouch
Bypassed Stomach
• Creates small stomach pouch
• Reroutes intestines
• Limits food intake & absorption
SLEEVE GASTRECTOMY
Portion Removed
• Removes part of the stomach
• Reduces stomach size
• Decreases hunger hormones
GASTRIC BAND
• Adjustable Band
Port Connecting to Port
• Adjustable silicone band
• Restricts food intake
• Reversible procedure
BILIARY PANCREATIC DIVERSION WITH DUODENAL SWITCH (BPD/DS)
Sleeve Stomach
• Sleeve gastrectomy + intestinal bypass
• Reduces absorption of calories
• Significant weight loss
BENEFITS OF SURGERY
• Major Weight Loss
• Improved Health
• Resolves Diabetes & More

- Has my weight significantly affected my health?

2. Learn about options

Understand:

- Benefits
- Risks
- Long-term commitment

3. Consider readiness

Think about:

- Willingness to follow long-term changes

4. Discuss with your doctor

If appropriate:

- Ask about eligibility
- Understand expectations

5. Keep a balanced perspective

Recognize:

- Surgery is one option among many

Chapter 13

Preventing Weight Regain: Protecting Your Progress

For many people, losing weight is only part of the journey.

Keeping it off is often the harder part.

Patients frequently tell me:

"Doctor, I can lose weight, but I always gain it back."

This is a very common and very frustrating experience.

If this has happened to you, you are not alone.

And more importantly, it does not mean you have failed.

Why Weight Regain Happens

After weight loss, the body does not simply accept the new weight.

It often responds in ways that favor weight regain.

You may notice:

- Increased hunger
- Stronger cravings
- Reduced metabolism

These are natural responses.

The body is trying to return to its previous weight.

At the same time, life continues:

- Busy schedules
- Stress
- Social events
- Old habits

All of these factors together make weight regain more likely.

The Subtle Nature of Regain

Weight regain usually happens gradually.

It often begins with small changes:

- Slightly larger portions
- Occasional extra snacks
- Reduced activity
- Less attention to habits

These changes may seem minor.

But over time, they add up.

That is why early awareness is so important.

Maintenance Requires a Shift in Thinking

Many people approach weight loss as a temporary effort.

They follow a plan, reach a goal, and then relax.

But maintenance requires a different mindset.

Weight management is ongoing.

It is not something you finish.

It is something you continue.

This does not mean constant struggle.

It means maintaining awareness and consistency.

Continue the Habits That Worked

The habits that helped you lose weight are the same ones that help you maintain it.

These include:

- Balanced eating
- Portion awareness
- Regular physical activity

- Adequate sleep

When these habits fade, weight regain becomes more likely.

The Role of Physical Activity

Physical activity becomes even more important during maintenance.

It helps:

- Burn calories
- Maintain muscle
- Support metabolism

Many people who successfully maintain weight loss stay physically active.

The goal is not intensity.

The goal is consistency.

Monitor Without Obsession

Monitoring helps detect changes early.

This may include:

- Weighing yourself once a week
- Noticing how clothes fit
- Observing eating patterns

Monitoring is not about anxiety.

It is about awareness.

Recognize Early Warning Signs

Pay attention to small changes:

- Increasing portion sizes
- More frequent snacking
- Reduced activity
- Less structured eating

If you notice these early, you can make small corrections before weight regain becomes significant.

Plan for Setbacks

Setbacks are part of life.

There will be times when:

- You eat more than planned
- Activity decreases
- Weight increases slightly

This is normal.

What matters is how you respond.

Instead of giving up:

- Return to your routine

- Reinforce your habits
- Move forward

Avoid All-or-Nothing Thinking

A common mistake is thinking:

"I gained a few pounds, so I have failed."

This mindset leads to:

- Frustration
- Loss of motivation
- Abandoning good habits

A better approach is:

- Accept small fluctuations
- Focus on long-term trends
- Stay consistent

Build a Simple Routine

Routine reduces the need for constant decision-making.

For example:

- Regular meal times
- Planned activity
- Consistent sleep schedule

A structured routine supports long-term success.

Stay Connected to Your Goals

Over time, it is easy to forget why you started.

Reconnect with your reasons:

- Better health
- More energy
- Improved mobility
- Greater independence

These reasons help maintain motivation.

Seek Support When Needed

You do not have to do this alone.

Support can come from:

- Healthcare providers
- Family and friends
- Support groups

Staying connected can help you stay accountable and encouraged.

When Additional Help Is Needed

If weight regain becomes significant, do not ignore it.

Early action is important.

Options may include:

- Revisiting lifestyle strategies
- Adjusting medications
- Seeking medical advice

Addressing the problem early prevents further regain.

A Long-Term Perspective

Weight management is not about perfection.

It is about maintaining a healthier pattern over time.

There will be fluctuations.

That is normal.

What matters is the overall direction.

Looking Ahead

In the final chapter, we will bring everything together.

We will create a clear, practical, long-term plan that you can follow with confidence.

Main Points to Remember

- Weight regain is common and expected
- The body tends to resist long-term weight loss
- Small changes can gradually lead to regain
- Maintenance requires ongoing attention
- Healthy habits must continue
- Physical activity is especially important
- Monitoring helps detect changes early
- Setbacks are normal and manageable
- Avoid all-or-nothing thinking
- Long-term consistency is key

What You Can Do Now

1. Monitor regularly

- Weigh yourself weekly
- Observe your habits

2. Identify risk areas

Ask:

- When am I most likely to slip?

3. Maintain activity

- Keep moving daily

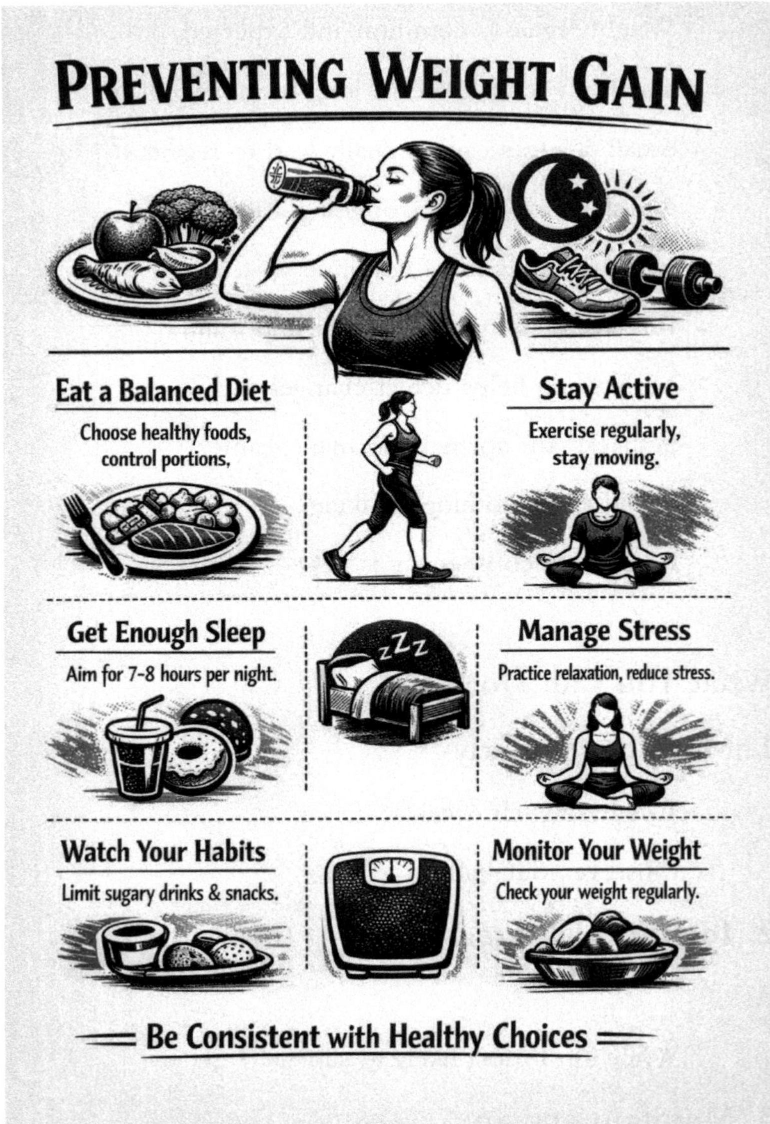
PREVENTING WEIGHT GAIN
Eat a Balanced Diet
Choose healthy foods, control portions.
Stay Active
Exercise regularly, stay moving.
Get Enough Sleep
Aim for 7-8 hours per night.
Manage Stress
Practice relaxation, reduce stress.
Watch Your Habits
Limit sugary drinks & snacks.
Monitor Your Weight
Check your weight regularly.
Be Consistent with Healthy Choices

4. Plan for setbacks

- Decide how you will respond

5. Stay consistent

Focus on:

- Long-term habits

Chapter 14

Your Long-Term Strategy for Lifelong Weight Control

We began this journey with a simple but deeply important question:

"Why can't I lose weight?"

Along the way, we explored many layers of that question.

You now understand:

- What obesity really is
- How it develops over time
- Why the body resists weight loss
- The role of food, habits, emotions, and activity
- When medical treatments may be helpful
- How to prevent weight regain

Now we come to the most important part.

How do you take all of this and apply it to your daily life?

There Is No Perfect Plan

One of the most important lessons is this:

There is no perfect plan.

There is only a plan that works for you.

Each person's life is different:

- Daily schedule
- Food preferences
- Health conditions
- Responsibilities
- Energy levels

A plan that fits your life is far more effective than one that looks perfect on paper but is difficult to follow.

Focus on the Big Picture

Long-term success does not depend on a single decision.

It depends on patterns.

Your daily choices, repeated over time, shape your results.

Instead of asking:

"What should I do today to lose weight?"

A better question is:

"What can I do consistently over the next few months?"

This shift changes everything.

The Four Pillars of Long-Term Success

Let us bring everything together into four simple areas.

1. Eating Patterns

- Balanced meals
- Portion awareness
- Reduced processed foods

2. Physical Activity

- Regular movement
- Walking or similar activity
- Strength maintenance

3. Behavior and Habits

- Consistent routines
- Awareness of triggers
- Gradual change

4. Medical Support (When Needed)

- Medications

- GLP-1 therapy
- Surgical options

These pillars work best when combined.

Start Small, Build Gradually

You do not need to change everything at once.

In fact, trying to do too much often leads to failure.

Instead:

- Choose one or two changes
- Practice them consistently
- Build gradually

For example:

- Walk daily
- Reduce sugary drinks
- Improve sleep

Small steps create lasting progress.

Create a Simple Daily Structure

A simple routine reduces confusion.

For example:

Morning:

- Planned breakfast
- Light activity if possible

Daytime:

- Regular meals
- Avoid unnecessary snacking

Evening:

- Light dinner
- Avoid late-night eating

This structure does not need to be rigid.

It needs to be consistent.

Monitor with Awareness

Monitoring helps you stay on track.

This may include:

- Weekly weight checks
- Observing eating habits
- Noticing energy levels

Do not use these as judgment.

Use them as guidance.

Expect Challenges

Life will not always be predictable.

There will be:

- Busy periods
- Travel
- Stress
- Illness

During these times:

- Do your best
- Avoid extreme decisions
- Return to routine when possible

Consistency over time matters more than temporary disruptions.

Redefine Success

Success is not only a number on the scale.

It includes:

- Better health
- Improved energy
- Better mobility
- Greater confidence
- More control over habits

Recognizing these improvements helps maintain motivation.

Be Patient

Weight management takes time.

There will be:

- Slow progress
- Plateaus
- Occasional setbacks

This is normal.

What matters is persistence.

Avoid Quick Fixes

Be cautious of:

- Extreme diets
- Miracle solutions
- Unrealistic promises

These approaches often lead to temporary results.

Sustainable change is more reliable.

Stay Connected to Your Purpose

Your reasons for wanting to lose weight are important.

They may include:

- Improving health
- Preventing disease
- Increasing energy
- Living more actively

These reasons provide direction.

Revisit them when motivation decreases.

Seek Support

You do not have to do this alone.

Support can come from:

- Healthcare providers
- Family
- Friends

Sharing your journey helps maintain accountability.

A Final Thought

Over many years of practice, I have seen a clear pattern.

People who succeed are not those who are perfect.

They are those who:

- Stay consistent

- Learn from setbacks
- Continue moving forward

You do not need to transform your life overnight.

You need to take one step, then another, and keep going.

This Is Your Journey

This book is not the end.

It is the beginning of a more informed and realistic approach.

You now understand the problem more clearly.

You have the tools to move forward.

And most importantly, you have the ability to make change.

It may not be fast.

It may not be perfect.

But it is possible.

Main Points to Remember

- There is no single perfect plan
- Long-term success depends on consistent habits
- Focus on eating, activity, behavior, and medical support when needed
- Small changes lead to meaningful results

- Monitoring helps maintain awareness
- Challenges are normal
- Success includes health and quality of life
- Patience and persistence are essential
- Avoid quick fixes
- Support improves long-term success

What You Can Do Now

1. Choose your starting point

Pick one or two changes:

- Improve diet
- Increase activity

2. Create a simple routine

Keep it realistic.

3. Set a short-term goal

For example:

- Follow your plan for one week

4. Track your progress

Notice:

- Habits
- Energy

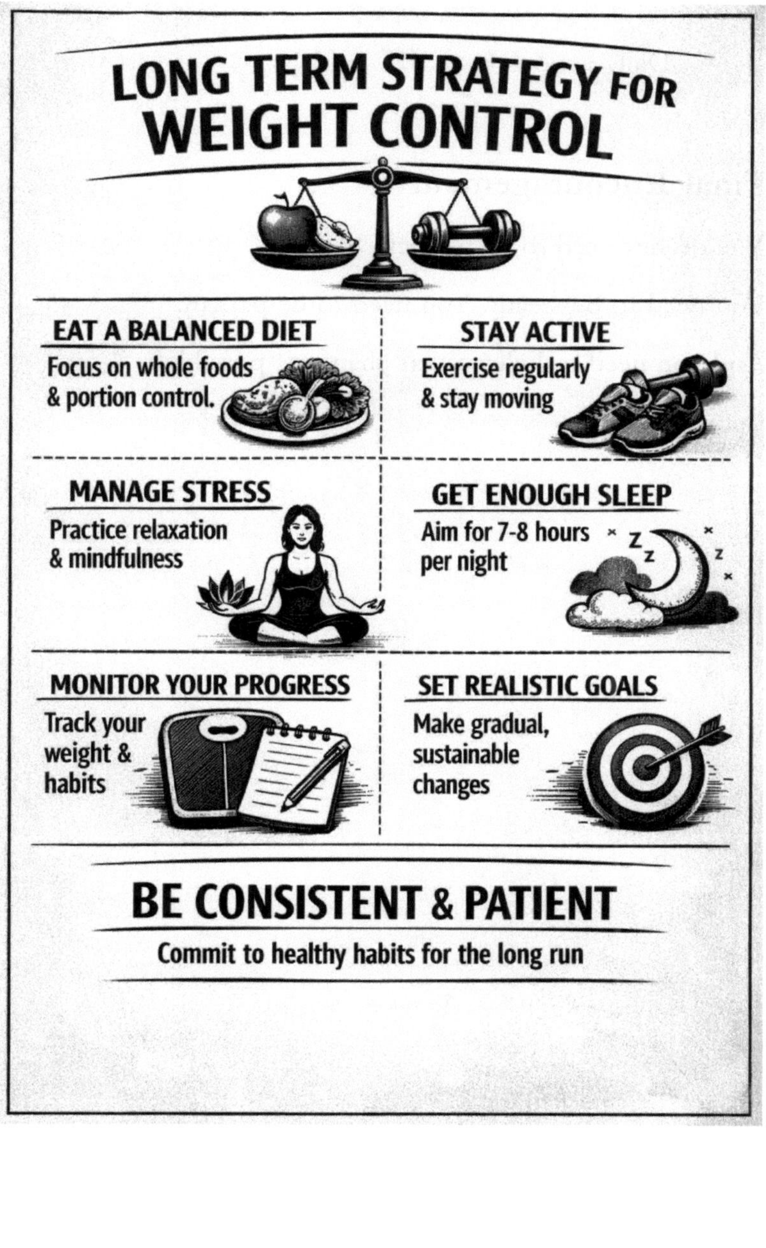
LONG TERM STRATEGY FOR WEIGHT CONTROL
EAT A BALANCED DIET
Focus on whole foods & portion control.
STAY ACTIVE
Exercise regularly & stay moving
MANAGE STRESS
Practice relaxation & mindfulness
GET ENOUGH SLEEP
Aim for 7-8 hours per night
MONITOR YOUR PROGRESS
Track your weight & habits
SET REALISTIC GOALS
Make gradual, sustainable changes
BE CONSISTENT & PATIENT
Commit to healthy habits for the long run

5. Stay consistent

Focus on:

- Daily actions

Final Encouragement

You do not need to be perfect.

You need to be steady. You need to be patient.

And you need to believe that change is possible.

Because it is.

Thank You and Please Review the Book

Thank you for taking the time to read this book. I sincerely hope it has helped you understand your health a little more clearly and has given you practical, everyday steps you can follow with confidence. If you found this book helpful, **I would truly appreciate it if you could leave a brief and honest review.** Even a few lines sharing your experience can make a meaningful difference. Your feedback helps other readers find reliable, trustworthy health information and supports them in making better decisions for themselves and their families.

Warm regards,

Dr Prabhat Das

Continue your Healthcare Journey

Good health is a journey, not a single step. It is not achieved in one day or with one book. That is why I created the **"Better Health with Dr Das"** series, with each book addressing a different common condition. If you would like easy, practical guidance on other everyday health concerns, you may wish to explore the rest of books in this series.

Books in this series:

- A Doctor's Easy Guide to Understanding & Managing **OBESITY**.

- A Doctor's Easy Guide to Understanding & Managing **HIGH BLOOD PRESSURE**.

- Doctor, What **DIET** Is Best for Me?

- Doctor, Why Can't I **Lose Weight?**

(a Doctor's Guide to safe & Sustainable Weight Loss)

- A Doctor's Easy Guide to **GLP-1 for Obesity**

- A Doctor's Guide to Living Well With **DIABETES**
- A Doctor's Guide to Understanding & Managing **HIGH CHOLESTEROL**

Printed by Libri Plureos GmbH in Hamburg, Germany

9 781971 672380